Human Communication

The Matrix of Nursing

Margaret L. Pluckhan, R.N., Ph.D.

Nursing Consultant
Colorado Department of Health

McGRAW-HILL BOOK COMPANY
A Blakiston Publication

New York St. Louis San Francisco Auckland Bogotá Düsseldorf
Johannesburg London Madrid Mexico Montreal New Delhi
Panama Paris São Paulo Singapore Sydney Tokyo Toronto

Notice

Medicine is an ever-changing science. As new research and clinical experience broaden our knowledge, changes in treatment and drug therapy are required. The editors and the publisher of this work have made every effort to ensure that the drug dosage schedules herein are accurate and in accord with the standards accepted at the time of publication. Readers are advised, however, to check the product information sheet included in the package of each drug they plan to administer to be certain that changes have not been made in the recommended dose or in the contraindications for administration. This recommendation is of particular importance in regard to new or infrequently used drugs.

Human Communication: The Matrix of Nursing

1 2 3 4 5 6 7 8 9 0 D O D O 7 8 3 2 1 0 9 8 7

This book was set in Times Roman by Creative Book Services, subsidiary of McGregor & Werner, Inc. The editor was Mary Ann Richter; the cover was designed by Scott Chelius; the production supervisor was Jeanne Selzam.
R. R. Donnelley & Sons Company was printer and binder.

Library of Congress Cataloging in Publication Data

Pluckhan, Margaret L
    Human communication.

    "A Blakiston publication."
    Includes bibliographies and index.
    1. Communication in nursing. 2. Inter-
personal communication. I. Title. [DNLM:
1. Communication. 2. Nurse-Patient relations.
WY87 P733h]
RT23.P54   301.14'02'4613   77-23966
ISBN 0-07-050352-4

Contents

074677

v

Part II
Human Communication Concepts, Principles, and Methodologies Applied to Nursing   135

Preface

Man is a socializing animal and has a basic need to relate to other human beings. It is as essential for man to communicate as it is for him to breathe. We cannot *not* communicate with others, yet when we attempt to communicate we often find that the relationships are impaired, rather than facilitated, by the interaction.*

Human communication is the process whereby we generate and transmit meaning. Communication is considered to be effective if the intended meaning of the sender is, at least to some degree, congruent with the meaning perceived by the receiver. Both the receiver and the sender of messages are continuously active participants in the process and are equally responsible for matching message meaning.

Frequently the human communication process is presented as a simple mechanistic flow of messages sent by verbal and nonverbal means across a

*The author wishes to convey to the reader the fact that efforts, although unsuccessful, were made to find an appropriate neuter pronoun for use throughout the writing of this book. Nonsexist references are to be inferred even though "he," "man," and other of the yet conventional masculine pronouns are used. Gender pronouns that have been used are to be considered as referring to persons of both or either sex.

variety of channels from one person to another. This conveyor belt or computer orientation to the complex process is totally inadequate. It fails to accommodate the human behavior that is *the* critical variable in the process. The process is indeed complex, dynamic, transactional and highly unpredictable. This is not to say that we must take communication behavior as it comes and do nothing to improve it. There are ways we can improve our odds in the "communication gamble," but they are not simplistic and predictable formulas or "how-to-do" schemes.

The author believes that we can improve our communication with self and others in three essential ways: (1) by increasing our appreciation and understanding of the process itself, (2) by increasing our understanding of self and fostering our own personal growth, and (3) by improving our sensitivity to others. The content of this book has been developed to address those three objectives. Concepts and principles relating to the human communication process are presented in Part I, together with an intrapersonal communication model that serves as a focal point for the study. Methods of general semantics, which have been applied to a variety of disciplines, including law, education, and medicine, are presented as a descriptive and prescriptive modality for application to nursing practice.

Part II of the book is devoted to the pragmatic application of the concepts and principles presented in the first section to a number of functional areas of nursing practice. Communication is the means by which we present ourselves to the world. It is the *matrix,* the glue or bond, for all life's activities and the essential ingredient of all nursing functions. Only a limited number of these functional areas could be presented. Those areas chosen are not to be considered the most important by any means. It is hoped that the reader will be able to make appropriate application of the content to other nursing activities.

Nursing, as a human service, relies heavily on the interpersonal communication and relationships that are established between the professional and the client and among members of the health team and the public. Tangential to our desire to improve the quality of health care must be our concerted effort to improve our communication skills. The study of the art and science of human communication is an exciting and challenging one that can pay high dividends to us personally and professionally.

This book is intended primarily as a textbook for nursing students and a practical reference for in-service coordinators, administrators, continuing education directors, and other nursing personnel. Increasing numbers of professional nursing programs are incorporating communication theory into their clinical and functional courses. Some programs have a basic communication course as a requirement in their curricula. The content and method of presentation of the material in this book lend themselves to either curriculum design. The first section of the book contains *basic* communication theory and methodologies that are appropriate and applicable to all disciplines and individuals.

ACKNOWLEDGMENTS

To my family, colleagues, and friends, who provided those essential ingredients of interest, support, and encouragement needed by any author to undertake a project of this kind

To the thousands of students whom I have had the pleasure of teaching and who in turn have been my teachers

To my mentors—the late Dr. William S. Middleton, who imprinted upon me a truly humanitarian approach to health care by his example, and Dr. Elwood Murray, whose excitement and enthusiasm for the field of speech communication generated that same spark of interest in me

To all the *significant others* who have played a part in developing my *frame of reference* by influencing the thoughts and feelings that are reflected in this manuscript

My sincere thanks
Margaret L. Pluckhan

Part 1

Basic Concepts, Theories, Principles, and Methodologies of Human Communication

Although this book is directed toward human communication as it applies to the nursing profession, the content presented in Part I is basic. It is germane to all individuals in both their personal and their professional lives, irrespective of their professional affiliation.

A brief overview of the history and genesis of the interdisciplinary nature of the field of human communication is presented. The intrapersonal human communication model, which was developed from a humanistic theory of the process of communication, serves as the framework for the content of the entire manuscript. The study of human communication is a study of human behavior and human relationships. The nervous system directs our unique and complex communication patterns.

In Part I, attention is drawn to man's unique and intriguing ability to symbolize, to represent to others through verbal and nonverbal language the world he has created. It is, to a large extent, the result of the use of capriciously and arbitrarily assigned symbols to convey meaning that disagreement in message meaning between individuals occurs. It is paradoxical that while effective communication calls for similarity in meaning between the sender and the receiver of messages, the very differences in meaning are what make interpersonal communication necessary and desirable. It would be a bland and lonely world indeed if everyone perceived and symbolized the world in the same way! There would be no need for individuals to get together to explore, discuss, debate, and resolve differences or to learn from one another.

Some of the potential external barriers and limiting internal factors that render our intrapersonal and interpersonal communication ineffective are presented in Part I. Dysfunctional communication results from the way in which we perceive ourselves, our perceptive defenses, the symbols we select, and assumptions we make. Further problems result from our overzealous concentration on verbal language at the expense of attending to the equally important nonverbal aspects of communication. Suggestions are presented for bridging some of the identified problems of communication.

When studying the human communication process, one cannot avoid learning more about one's own unique behavior; one's thought, perceptual, and symbolic processes and patterns of behaving with others. Our verbal and nonverbal language serve not only as a means of communication but also as a diagnostic tool relating to the functioning of our nervous system and sense organs. All of the areas mentioned will be discussed in Part I.

Chapter I

Introduction

The longer I live the more do human beings appear to be fascinating and full of interest . . .
Maxim Gorki

Just as we become better informed about an individual by learning about his origins and background experiences, so we may shed light on the field of human communication through a brief history of its development. The study of human communication had its genesis in the field of rhetorical communication, which deals primarily with the rules of good speechmaking and the art and science of debate. Rhetoric has been recognized as such for thousands of years. In fact, the oldest known essay dates back to 3000 B.C. and gives advice on how to speak effectively.[1] The traditional emphasis in speech departments across the country has been and in many

---

[1]James C. McCroskey, *An Introduction to Rhetorical Communication*, 2d ed., Prentice-Hall, Englewood Cliffs, N.J., 1972, p. 3.

cases remains public address, the art and science of inquiry, argumentation, and persuasion. Major attention is focused on content and on the performance of the sender or message source.

Studying rhetoric involves gaining skill in techniques and methods of persuasion. Particular attention is directed toward the conception and organization of an idea, selection of appropriate words and phrases, delivery, and continuity. These procedural steps are known as the five classical *canons of rhetoric* and are labeled *invention, disposition, style, memory,* and *delivery.* Rhetoricians are concerned with the credibility or image of the speaker (*ethos*), the emotion and response of the audience (*pathos*), and the nature of the message and its delivery to the audience (logos). Rhetoric and debate courses, which include concepts and theories from such disciplines as political science, philosophy, logic, English, history, economics, and, more recently, the behavioral sciences, are generally a part of the curriculum for lawyers and clergy. The traditional field of rhetoric has been slowly changing over the years and is showing increased acceptance of and interest in the behavioral aspects of speech, the nonverbal as well as the verbal aspects.

HISTORY OF SPEECH COMMUNICATION

Our present-day study of human communication is found under the rubric of "speech communication" and goes beyond the traditional formal speechmaking process. It includes a more comprehensive and pragmatic approach to the informal social interactions of everyday life. In fact, human communication theorists and methodologists have been referred to as "social science technicians" and "social engineers." Human communication is a relatively new yet rapidly evolving field of study. Ogden and Richards were pioneers in the field. Their book *The Meaning of Meaning* was first published in 1923 and dealt with the influence of language upon thought and the science of symbolism.[2] Its focus was *semantics,* or how language or any kind of discourse produces understanding in an audience. Richards is considered to be the first major communication theorist in the modern sense.

In 1933 a significant contribution to the communication field was made by Alfred Korzybski, with his book *Science and Sanity: An Introduction to Non-Aristotelian Systems and General Semantics.*[3] He provided a description of the psychological implications of language and its effect on man.

[2]C. K. Ogden and I. A. Richards, *The Meaning of Meaning,* Harcourt, Brace & World, New York, 1923.

[3]Alfred Korzybski, *Science and Sanity: An Introduction to Non-Aristotelian Systems and General Semantics,* 4th ed., The International Non-Aristotelian Library Publishing Co., Lakeville, Conn., 1958.

General semantics, the study of the relationship between language, thought, and behavior, was presented as a prescriptive tool for preventing and correcting dysfunctional communication. More detailed discussion of principles of general semantics will be presented in Chapter 7. Korzybski acknowledged a relationship between language and personality and subsequently between personality and speech disorders.

Concepts and theories from the more established disciplines, such as psychology, sociology, anthropology, and cybernetics, began to be recognized as both relevant and essential to the study of man the communicator. By the 1940s *human communication* as a discrete field of study was offered in speech departments at many universities and colleges across the country. The substance of the courses bore little resemblance to content offered in the traditional field of speech—rhetoric and debate. Human communication is both an art and a science. It is the study of the complex information processing system of man and the means by which humans link themselves with one another and with the world.

At the 1968 New Orleans Conference on Research and Instructional Development, "speech-communication"* was adopted as the label to reflect the efforts made toward maintaining a marriage between the traditional speech field and the human communication field within the Speech Association of America. While speech communication referred primarily to *spoken symbolic interactions,* the significance of nonverbal aspects of communication was also recognized. Theory and research about nonverbal behavior were late in developing and consequently lacked sophistication at that time. However, increasing attention is now being directed toward understanding the meaning of messages from body movement (kinesics), man's use of space (proxemics), and man's territorial drives.

While traditional speech and human communication have been placed under the umbrella of speech communication, they involve concepts and methodologies that place them a world apart. A major difference is that rhetorical communication is concerned with logic and proof, usually in a formal setting, while human communication focuses on interpersonal conflict and resolution in the informal everyday situation. In traditional speechmaking, greater emphasis is placed on the speaker (message source) and on a one-way person-to-group transfer of message, in contrast with human communication, in which equal attention, importance, and responsibility are assigned to the sender *and* the receiver of messages. In rhetoric, rules and prescribed procedures are laid down, whereas in human communication the need to understand the complex human process, the uniqueness of individuals, and the inappropriateness of distinct techniques or procedures for improving the odds of matching meaning are emphasized.

*The hyphen was later dropped, and the group became known as the Speech Communication Association of America.

Possibly the most obvious difference is that the rhetorician uses Aristotelian theory while the communication theorist in general and the general semanticist in particular subscribe to a non-Aristotelian methodology for ridding the system of dysfunctional communication.

Research in human communication relies more heavily on controlled laboratory experimentation, while research in rhetoric depends more on field observation. Both fields are concerned with application and experiential learning through feedback and have the overall goal of manipulating and controlling man's thoughts and actions. This goal is not to be viewed as a detrimental activity but rather as the interpersonal influence essential for man's survival. While the theory of rhetoric may have been the base upon which the field of human communication was developed, the theoretical and methodological differences of the two fields are readily apparent.

WHAT IS HUMAN COMMUNICATION?

Human communication is the *generation and transmission of meaning,* not a simple transfer of verbal and nonverbal messages from sender to receiver as is so often assumed. The focus of concern is the production of *meaning*, not messages. Human communication is the process of eliciting responses to stimuli. Any person, object, event, or activity that stimulates a perception and a response in a person results in communication. There is no communication if the stimulus is ignored. The stimulus may be intentional or unintentional, and the receiver may be aware or totally unaware of his response to it. In fact, many of our messages (stimuli) are sent and received below the level of awareness of any of those directly involved in the process. It is also common for some responses to be largely intrapsychic, with only a subtle overt response noted.

Intrapersonal communication is the process that occurs *within* the individual himself whereby meaning is generated. The stimulus may originate internally, such as with hunger pains or other physiological stimuli, or from external sources, such as a sound coming from the environment. *Interpersonal* communication, on the other hand, involves a transaction *between* two or more individuals. Dyadic, intragroup, intergroup, and multigroup communication would be examples of interpersonal communication. Intrapersonal and interpersonal communication and their relationship will be discussed in more detail in subsequent chapters.

We cannot transmit meaning, as such, to others. We can only transmit stimuli in the form of words and actions, through which associations can be made by the other individual and subsequently take on unique meaning. Nothing has meaning in and of itself, but any stimulus can serve as a potential source for eliciting meaning and response in an individual. Each person invents and assigns meaning to stimuli in his unique and unlimited way, as he makes his own reality.

While communication occurs when a stimulus generates meaning in an individual, *effective* communication requires the message meaning intended by the sender and the meaning generated in the receiver to be *isomorphic* or at least to bear some resemblance to one another. The attempt to attain effective communication is directed toward matching meaning, toward gaining consistency and approaching congruence between intended message meaning and received meaning. A perfect match of meaning is virtually impossible for humans to attain. This fact will become increasingly obvious as the multitude of variables and complexities of the human communication process are discussed. We are constantly being confronted by new and different situations, varied environmental settings, and a galaxy of unique individuals. Miscommunication under those conditions is not only common but to be expected. Some individuals are less adept than others as communicators. A fact that all must accept is that we may have a high degree of success in attaining effective communication at certain times but become totally inadequate with other individuals and/or in other situations. As Abraham Lincoln once said, "Even a dog cannot reach all of the fleas." But even like the dog, we do not quit trying. In fact, the difficulty of the task should provide us with a true incentive and a worthwhile challenge, for the payoff is immeasurable.

Human communication is not a language process, as is so often thought, but a *people* process and a *social* process. The generation and transmission of meaning reside in people, not in words or messages. Each person produces meaning that makes sense to him from the stimulus received. Linguistic skills are not to be equated with communication skills. We acquire the ability to speak early in life, but communicative effectiveness is only a relative thing throughout our lifetime. The most melodious and eloquent words are only vain sounds if we cannot comprehend or attach the intended meaning to them.

We are a verbal society. The verbal utterances we experience every day are deafening. But the use of verbal language, although our principal means of communication, is not the only means we have. There are innumerable *nonverbal* stimuli with the power to generate meaning, not the least of these being the spatial and temporal dimensions. Touch and smoke signals were some of our most primitive forms of communication, and they generally were more effective than the sophisticated spoken and written words we use today.

A distinction must be made between "communication" and "communications." Communications refers to the technical means by which messages are sent. Television, radio, telephone, and the newspaper are examples of instruments or media through which communication may flow. The focus of this book is on communication, or the human process of eliciting meaning.

PURPOSE OF COMMUNICATION

All communication has purpose, the overall intent being to *influence* or *persuade*. Through our thought processes and fantasy, we persuade ourselves as well as others. For example, we may "psych ourselves out" and thereby convince ourselves of our own ability to perform a Herculean task. Our unused potential can be activated through intrapersonal communication and influence. We expend a great deal of our energies trying to impress others and convince them of our worth through devious as well as obvious means. Even our *phatic communication*, the "Hi, how are you?" is an attempt to influence others by getting their attention and then checking to determine whether the psychological climate is conducive to interpersonal communication and influence. Phatic communication serves to bring individuals together and thereby exerts interpersonal influence. Through speech we exercise influence on society. By banding together into groups to fight a cause, we can exert sufficient influence to bring about change. As we communicate information, we have the potential to influence others to modify their behavior.

Some communication theorists claim that the purpose of communication is twofold: to get *pleasure* as well as to control or influence. This notion seems logical in view of the fact that man is a social animal and pursues many pleasurable experiences through interpersonal encounters.

Another major purpose of communication, which may be tangential to both influence and pleasure, is *survival*. As we lose influence over our external environment, we resign ourselves to isolation and the pathological behavior and death that result. All systems, whether individuals, groups, or complex organizations, require continual inputs if they are to survive. Individually we cannot maintain emotional stability for prolonged periods of time when communicating only with self. *Entropy* is the term used in thermodynamics to identify a system that is closed to new inputs and eventually dies.

HUMAN COMMUNICATION AS PROCESS

Human communication is a complex, transactional, and dynamic process; a circular, continuous, essential, and irreversible series of actions. It is therefore not too surprising that it is also highly unpredictable. It is not a simple procedure or series of events that are easily understood and for which skill can be readily and permanently developed. The parameters are broad, the variables are infinite, and a degree of uncertainty is inevitable.

The question is, Where and how does one approach the study of such a complex process? A fragmented approach focusing on isolated incidents and parts of the total process would provide a false picture, yet to study and present the total system as a gestalt is overwhelming. The answer to the dilemma seems to reside in the reader, who must remain constantly aware of the interrelationship among the variables in the process. A chance remark cannot be fully understood or explained when taken out of context. Few insights have been gained from research into isolated incidents or segments of the process. It is as impractical to fragment the process for study as it is to explain the process of transportation of our drinking water by simply describing the mechanism in the faucet handle.

Superficially the statement "All I want to know is how to say what I mean and to know others understand it" seems to be a very simple request. However, it is not simple when one recognizes the multitude of interrelated factors that must be considered. The communication process is a *complex* system that involves unique human internal systems interacting in specific situations and in particular settings or environments. There is no distinct cause/effect relationship, no either/or situation or expected behavior. To understand human communication behavior we must learn about the nature of man and of society. Yet human factors operating in the sender and receiver and in the relationship are often unknown and/or poorly understood. For example, a great deal of mystery remains about the perceptual and cognitive processes of man. For the time being, we must resign ourselves to the use of the *black Box concept** as we attempt a comprehensive study of the complex communication process.

Human communication is not a mechanical stimulus-response reaction, not an interaction with something or someone, but a *transaction*. There is a reciprocating influence among variables. Each aspect of the process bears a relationship to each other aspect. Just as in family therapy there is no one isolated family member identified as "client," so there is no one isolated variable in the communication system of that family. A global and comprehensive approach again is required in explaining and understanding this transactional process.

In the communication process we are dealing not with a simple mixture of elements but with a complex compound that is more than the sum of its parts. It is analogous to the chemical effect of codeine and aspirin: the effect of each of these drugs taken alone differs from the synergistic effect that results when they are taken together.

*A term used in cybernetics to signify that something, yet unknown, in its operational details happens.

The human communication process is *dynamic*: fluid and ever-changing from moment to moment. People change; situations and settings change. Our communication events cannot be situationally or intrapsychically replicated for study. No two situations are exactly alike, nor does one's internal system remain in a static state whereby similar message meaning might be expected over time. This fact is readily evident when we use a particular approach with an individual one day and get one kind of response, use the same approach the following day and get a totally different reaction. No two individuals ever have the identical experience, nor does one person ever have the exact same experience twice. "We never walk in the same river" is a common expression. The water, rocks, banks, debri, and people all change as we walk in that river. Even artificial flowers exhibit some change: they gather dust and/or fade. The variables that affect our communication with self and others are as fluid and evasive as the mercury from a broken thermometer we try to retrieve from the floor.

Human communication is a *circular* process with neither a discrete beginning nor an ending. As such, each individual in the interchange simultaneously acts as a sender and a receiver of messages and a generator of meaning. While a diagram depicting a one-way flow of information from sender to receiver may be appropriate for explaining computers and practical as a representation of the communication process, it is inadequate and misleading.

As a process, human communication is a *continuous* series of actions toward some end. Humans are in almost continuous communication with one another and transmit and generate meaning in many ways. Intrapersonal communication, as we communicate with self in fantasy, thought, and dream, consumes much of our time.

The communication process is *irreversible*. We cannot *un*communicate or take back a message once sent. In addition, the information that is stored in our efficient memory bank is always available for future interactions. Man differs from lower animals in his unique ability to bind time. *Time-binding* provides man with the capacity to preserve and retrieve the past. This unique ability obviously has both beneficial and detrimental effects. It may prevent us from repeating a previous mistake but also prevents us from retrieving words or actions. "I forgive you for saying that" is only a rhetorical statement. Errors rooted in language are indeed difficult to erase. The nurse who chooses to do "desk work," to work with papers, rather than relate to people may be fully aware of the fact that while mistakes made on paper can be more easily corrected, those made by the spoken word to staff or clients immediately become a permanent part of future interactions. It is as impossible to retrieve words once spoken as it is to put toothpaste back into the tube.

Human communication is a gamble, a game of chance. The uncertain and highly *unpredictable* nature of the process is primarily due to the process's dynamic quality and the complexity of the variables—some yet unknown. We gamble not only that the message stimuli we send will elicit some meaning and response from another individual, but even more important, that the intended meaning will be, to a degree, in harmony with the message meaning generated. While a 100 percent probability of attaining effective communication is unrealistic, we may have to be content with even a 50 percent chance of success. In fact, it has been estimated that we have *effective* communication only about 35 percent of the time. With such low odds, one generally would refuse to bet or take the risk or play the game. It is ironic as well as frustrating to realize that we know where a star will be 5 years from now but cannot more accurately predict the communicative responses of rational man the next minute.

Even though human communication is a gamble with low odds of success, we cannot refuse to engage ourselves in its activities. Communication is *essential* to life in a civilized society. Through interpersonal influence we control our environment and ensure our survival. We cannot not communicate. Even when we refrain from sending word messages, our body language sends messages that have communication potential. Communication constitutes the core of culture and indeed of life itself.

THE INTERDISCIPLINARY NATURE OF HUMAN COMMUNICATION

The field of human communication has borrowed heavily from concepts, theories, and methodologies of the behavioral and social sciences, the humanities, and the physical sciences. Those applied from the traditional field of rhetoric have already been discussed. There is no *one* theory of human communication, but most of the theories proposed include substance from the fields of psychology, sociology, anthropology, linguistics, and cybernetics. Following is a discussion of a limited number of the related disciplines (Figure 1-1) and their contributions to human communication theory.

The field of *psychology* has contributed theories of personality and human behavior. Much of our understanding of man's thought and complex cognitive or perceptual processes has been derived from research findings in the area of psychology. These, together with theories about attitudes, feelings, and basic human needs, have been indispensible in the development of theories and models of intrapersonal communication. Psychologists have formulated innumerable theories of self-consistency that have aided our understanding of message selection and meaning generation. Psychological concepts have increased our knowledge of man

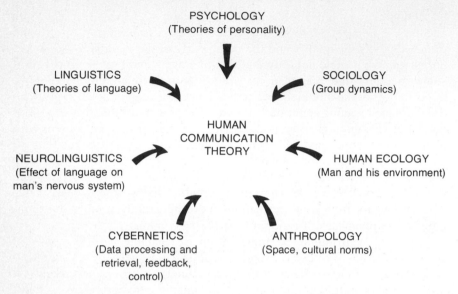

Figure 1-1   Interdisciplinary contributions to human communication theory.

as data processor and transformer. The interface between psychological theory and human communication theory is evident in the diagnosis and treatment of mental illness. Family therapy and psychotherapy are generally approached from the standpoint of failures in intrapersonal and interpersonal communication.

A discussion of human communication would be incomplete without at least some mention of what has been labeled *paranormal communication, psi,* or *the psychic phenomena* in the field of parapsychology. Extrasensory perception (ESP), telepathy, and clairvoyance are modes of communication that have been acclaimed as having much in common with *normal* communication. Over the years, increasing attention has been paid to psychic phenomena. The reader is encouraged to refer to a report of an entire research symposium related to paranormal communication, which is presented in the *Journal of Communication*.[4]

While psychology traditionally focuses on individual behavior, *sociology* concerns itself with the personality and dynamics of groups. Content areas relative to groups, together with theories of social order, status, and factors of social influence, contribute to our knowledge of interpersonal communication. A book of selected papers of Lewin, edited by Cartwright, is a classic in the field of sociology.[5] The book presents such concepts as

[4]"Paranormal Communication: A Research Symposium," *Journal of Communication,* **25**(1): 96–194, Winter 1975.

[5]Dorwin Cartwright (ed.), *Field Theory in Social Science: Selected Theoretical Papers by Kurt Lewin,* Harper & Row, Publishers, New York, 1951.

those of life space, social norms, norm formation, and role theory, all of which shed light on the constraints on communication behavior. Sociology has contributed theories concerning the democratic process and consensus in group problem solving and decision making which are most relevant to communication and information processing. The concepts from the social sciences which are appropriate, readily applicable, and essential to the development of human communication theory are numerous.

Through the study of *cultural anthropology,* the communication theorist has gained substantial knowledge of cultural and perceptual differences in cross-cultural communication behavior. Cultural variables, such as norms, customs, rituals, myths, traditions, and unique symbolic behavior, affect one's internal psychic system. Cultural components act as constraints on one's communication behavior and produce dysfunctional intercultural communication. The need to understand cultural differences becomes more urgent as past territorial boundaries are extended through rapid air and space travel. Hall referred to our dysfunctional communication across cultural lines when he said, "Most of our behavior does not spring from malice but from ignorance."[6] Hall went so far as to say, "Culture is communication and communication is culture."[7] He proposed that everything man is and does is associated with his experience in space. Hall's classic contribution to human communication theory has been in the area of nonverbal *proxemics*, or man's use of space, and the exploration into cultural differences in his use of space.

The contributions of another anthropologist, Robert Ardrey, are considered to be substantial. Reference to his theories and research findings will be made repeatedly throughout this book. Ardrey focused his attention on explaining *why* we use space, why we have a need to secure and defend territory.[8] The theory of *territoriality* offers a logical explanation for much of our nonverbal communication behavior and is appropriate to the study of social as well as physical space. Ardrey's theory of the triad of basic human needs for *identity, stimulation,* and *security* provides a logical explanation for much of the communication behavior of man. More detailed discussion of these basic human needs as they relate to communication theory will be presented in subsequent chapters.

An explanation for the relationship between man and his environment as well as greater understanding of the important process of symbolic transformation between man's internal and external environments come from the field of *human ecology.* As children we learn and program our system through interaction with our environment, and the permanent

[6]Edward T. Hall, *The Silent Language,* Fawcett Publications, Greenwich, Conn., 1959, p. 9.
[7]Hall, *The Silent Language,* p. 169.
[8]Robert Ardrey, *The Territorial Imperative,* Atheneum Publishers, New York, 1966.

imprint that results affects our communication behavior. Theories of adaptation, selectivity, and man's efforts to maintain some semblance of equilibrium are gleaned from the study of human ecology. The interface between human ecology and communication is evident when we realize that through communication behavior we are able to relate to our external environment and survive.

It is self-evident that *linguistics*, the science of language, is an essential part of communication theory. Language is acknowledged to be our major tool of human communication. Dialect and regional differences must be explored and considered if effective communication is our goal. It is imperative that we understand how the structure of our language affects man's nervous system and how that in turn relates to his communication behavior. Theories from the fields of *neurophysiology* and *neurolinguistics* are also involved. Insights into *organ language*, or how disease or physical illness sends out messages, are of particular concern to the study of human communication in the health field. Theories on the relationship between the emotions and physiological changes in the body have joined the fields of psychology and medicine in the further study of psychosomatic illness.

Man, like the computer, is a data processor. While there are striking differences between the unpredictable human processor and the highly predictable, mechanical machine, there are many concepts from the fields of *mathematics* and *cybernetics* which are appropriate to our human data processing system. Cybernetics is the science of communication and control. It is concerned with techniques for generating, gathering, storing, and retrieving ideas quickly and effectively. Theories relating to data processing, storage, feedback, and the mechanics of a self-regulating system used in cybernetics are equally relevant, with some modifications, to man the data processor. Some of the concepts of cybernetics, such as the black Box and entropy, have already been discussed. Others, such as noise and redundancy, will be presented later in the book.

These are but some of the theoretical contributions from other disciplines which have aided our knowledge and understanding of the complex human communication process. Research instruments used in the study of communication and methodologies appropriate to improving our communication skills can also be traced to these and other disciplines. It should be apparent that the study of human communication uses an eclectic approach.

THE IMPORTANCE OF HUMAN COMMUNICATION

To question the importance of communication in our personal, professional, and political lives would be as foolhardy as to question our need for air and water. Man is a social animal, and his very existence depends upon his ability to communicate with himself, with others, and with his environment. Living is basically communicating. We communicate to survive, to maintain and regain our sanity, to bring structure and organization into our lives, to control, and to gain pleasure. We seek out others and communicate with them because we cannot bear the pains of isolation. We engage in communication behavior virtually every minute of our waking and sleeping hours, in thoughts, in dreams, or in interpersonal relationships.

Through rapid air travel, nations have been brought closer together and our galaxy of interpersonal communication has been expanded. Cultural barriers that cause communication problems have to be dissolved. Détente reflects our efforts to reduce the potential of future wars between nations through effective communication at the conference table. The July 1975 hookup between American and Russian astronauts in space was largely a communication feat. Establishing and maintaining cooperation and effective communication were essential.

Dysfunctional communication is in evidence all around us. It warrants our concern, for it is costly. Our prejudices and biases, which are developed and expressed through the communication process, become a permanent part of our internal system and have propagated riots, international wars, and general social unrest.

Our sophisticated scientific advancement and technological achievements have communicated a false impression that nothing is impossible and that there are no limits to what can be achieved or what individuals can have. Many people, especially disturbed individuals, view reality through distorted filters and have gained an unrealistic notion of what they can expect out of life. Often they regress to the childlike behavior of not wanting to defer gratification and pleasure and insist on getting everything *now*. This utopian attitude eventually leads to disappointment and hostility, which frequently are communicated through outbursts of criminal activity. The fight for territory and possessions by individuals as well as by nations has led to crime, emotional stress, and bloodshed. Our jails and mental hospitals are filled with individuals who have been unable to communicate effectively in society. The number of hospital beds and clinic visits assigned to individuals suffering from psychological problems is but one index of the magnitude of the problem of misevaluation in our communication with self and others.

Mental illness has been identified as America's primary health problem, afflicting at least 10 percent of our population. Mental illness represents an economic drain of at least $21 billion a year. Psychopathology is a relationship problem often caused by dysfunctional intrapersonal and interpersonal communication. Schizophrenia, which accounts for most of the mental illness, is a communication defect. The schizophrenic individual has difficulty in interpersonal relationships, has problems with logical thought, often oversymbolizes, and has difficulty making even simple choices. Verbal exchange is a weak area for the person with a schizophrenic personality. Most neuroses and psychoses are diagnosed and the unconscious mental activities inferred from expressed communication from the client. The therapy for most mental illness focuses upon altering verbal behavior and ridding the ill system of *semantic bacteria*, or the linguistic pathogens that warp meaning. Efforts are made to encourage verbalization as a way to help the client reorganize his world. Communication theory and methodology are crucial to the study of mental illness, to its diagnosis as well as its treatment.

Psychological problems are social problems, individual problems are family problems, and all are communication problems. Communication is the bond that brings families together, keeps them together, or causes their members to drift apart. The increasing incidence of divorce, or our growing "marriage mortuary" as it has been called, can be attributed to dysfunctional communication among couples; and it threatens to destroy the substance of our family life.

Communication is important to us in the numerous ways already mentioned. In addition, we manage and control situations in our personal and social lives as we exert interpersonal influence through communication behavior. While our communication produces many problems, it also serves as the means by which we learn about ourselves and others and resolve problems in life. Each of us develops his own unique personality through association and communication with others. We reveal ourselves to others through our verbal utterances as well as by nonverbal means. "How do I know what I think until I hear what I say?" speaks to the point. It is through communication that we learn our personal identity. Demosthenes said, "As a vessel is known by the sound, whether it is cracked or no, so men are proved by their speeches whether they are wise or foolish." It conveys a similar message as the saying "Better to remain silent and be thought a fool than to speak out and remove all doubt." Efforts to improve our communication, to learn more about self and how we relate to others, are reflected in the increasing popularity of personal growth experience workshops and training sessions. Mental health means effective intrapersonal and interpersonal communication.

The title of this book, *Human Communication: The Matrix of Nursing,* reflects at least the biased notion of this author as to the importance of communication to the field of nursing. Human communication influences and molds the outcome of all nursing activities. Just as collagen holds us together physically or as mortar holds bricks together, so communication is the bond, glue, or matrix that is the essential substance for nursing functions. Nursing is a social process that involves data gathering and processing as well as interpersonal communication with clients, the public, nursing staff, students, and health team members as the nurse seeks to affect health care. Although it may be presumptuous to claim communication as the essential ingredient in *all* nursing activities, it is equally difficult to conceive of a single nursing activity that does not in some way involve communication. Effective communication has been identified as *the greatest single weakness in hospitals today*. There is no factor more vital to the goal of providing quality care than the relationship established between the nurse and the client, the nursing administrator and staff, or the faculty member and student. It has been said that the doctor has a human life in his hands, but there is a sense in which the nurse has much more: the protection, development, and care of a human personality. We assume this responsibility as we develop honest and open communication with others. Smith proposed that "the science of communication is more pertinent to nursing than the science of disease or pathology."[9]

The importance of interpersonal communication to health professionals themselves was evident from a *Denver Post* article that stated that the suicide rate among dentists was the highest rate of any profession. It was explained on the basis that dentists are trained primarily to be technicians and to work with tools rather than with people. They eventually found in practice that the teeth are connected to people who are in turn attached to emotions that are expressed, often emphatically, to the dentist, who is ill-equipped to deal with them. The frustrations and stresses are considered to be precursors to potential suicide. As have many medical schools today, schools of dentistry have included courses in human relations and communication in their curricula and are now giving more attention to the *people* behind the teeth or the illness.

While nursing curricula have generally included courses in the behavioral and social sciences, discrete course work in communication theory and methodologies would be an appropriate addition at all levels of study. All nurses engage in communication-related problem solving, data collection and processing, evaluation, management, teaching, and coordination. The part communication plays in these and other roles and responsibilities is presented in more detail in Part II.

WAYS TO ATTAIN EFFECTIVE COMMUNICATION

Man has two faults—what he *says* and what he *does*—and both involve communication. To reduce these human failings we obviously must do something about our communication behavior. Communication is a "game" we play our entire lifetime. It is neither innately nor intuitively

[9]Dorothy M. Smith, "Myth and Method in Nursing Practice," *American Journal of Nursing,* **64**(2):70, February 1964.

derived. It is a difficult game that must be learned. When a child first learns to talk, we are inclined to infer that he has now learned to communicate. Nothing is more contrary to fact. Communication is *not* synonymous with speaking, and in fact, talking at times is inversely related to the effectiveness of our communication behavior. We may talk rapidly and even eloquently yet fail to communicate.

Communication, unlike wine, does not improve with age. People often ask, "Why doesn't the man of 60 years who has spent 20 years in bed look more rested?" A similar question might be asked in relation to communication. We spend over 70 percent of our lives in communication activities, so why can't we expect a 60-year-old person who has spent 42 of those years communicating to do a better job of it? The open and honest communication of children becomes lost in adults, who use words to disguise and distort their true feelings so as to protect themselves from others and conform to social demands. Children do not feel the threat that adults learn to feel and do not have so great a need to please and impress others. I recall a pleasant, honest message I received from a child who passed me on the street one day as I was walking my dog. As the dog pulled on the lead and seemingly was gasping for breath, the child passed me and said, "Lady, you ought to walk faster. You're choking your dog!" An adult might have cloaked his true feelings by saying, "Your dog sure is taking *you* for a walk." As we respond to our programmed "should" and "should not" system, the honesty of children is dissipated and the effectiveness of our communication is lost along with it.

There are three basic ways by which we can improve our odds in the communication gamble. We can improve our rate of success in matching meaning by (1) increasing our appreciation and understanding of the communication process itself, (2) improving our awareness and understanding of self, and (3) becoming more sensitive to others.

Human communication is both a science and an art and therefore requires *knowledge of the concepts and theories of the process as well as skill in applying them*. Like giving an intramuscular injection, effective communication requires practice, time and effort, and a sincere desire to improve.

Communication skills are best learned *experientially*. Communication does not happen in a social vacuum. Effective communication cannot be learned except through interaction with others. This fact was evident from a study conducted using a programmed text in interpersonal relationships.[10] Senior students in a leadership course studied each of the 10

[10]Margaret Pluckhan, "A Study of the Effectiveness of the General Relationship Improvement Program through Its Use with a Selected Group of Students in Nursing," in *Toward More Effective Teaching in WCHEN Schools,* Western Interstate Commission for Higher Education, Boulder, Colo., 1964, pp. 25–26.

lessons of the text in dyads, interacting in pairs. Retention test scores 11 weeks after the sessions were completed revealed a surprising 92 percent retention of the material learned. These findings were particularly signficant when they were compared with the minimal retention rates that result from our conventional didactic methods of teaching and from other content areas. The encouraging results were explained on the basis of the rewarding effects of the programmed approach to learning. However, in retrospect an equally feasible explanation might be the superiority of the experiential learning that took place as the pairs learned about interpersonal relationships from interaction with one another.

We must all admit that we have spent comparatively little time in our personal and professional lives trying to prevent communication breakdown. Most often we are motivated by crisis situations rather than by prior planning. Unfortunately we begin to think about how a machine works only when it breaks down. The same can be said for learning about the communication process. We engage in a wide array of human relationships, but only when problems force us to find remedies do we try to understand what went on and make the necessary repairs. We can attend to only one thing at a time, and generally we are so busy with our performance of a task that we forget the important part communication plays in attaining that goal. Most of the problems relate to our verbal exchanges. It may be no coincidence that man's best friend does not talk!

We can improve our ability as communicators by gaining new knowledge, insights, and points of view. Some of the myths about communication must be explored, exposed, and exploded, especially the magical solutions and set formulas that guarantee success. For example, many of the traditional approaches to communication deal with the isolated subject of "listening." Such discussions often leave one with the false impression that if we concentrate on the sound waves and "open our ears," we will have success in communication. Listening is an active part of the entire complex perceptual process and involves more than auditory sensation. There are medicine men with gimmicks and patent drugs who claim to cure all communication ills. It behooves all of us to be skeptical of any prescribed, simplistic, mechanistic, or foolproof remedies to communication problems. Individuals who look for simplistic answers are like Don Quixote, the idealistic and impractical hero of Cervantes, batting at windmills and serving only to frustrate himself.

The first way to improve our communication is to gain knowledge. General semantics as a descriptive and prescriptive field of study of man's reaction to language provides valuable insights but proclaims no singular and final answer. These and other methodologics will be discussed throughout this book. Many of the black Boxes, or voids, in our knowledge can be filled through research studies in communication and related fields.

Some of the most commonly used measuring instruments are the Osgood Semantic Differential for the study of individual behavior, the Galvanic Skin Response, and the Bales Interaction Process Analysis for the study of task and process functions and verbal and nonverbal behavior in groups. Moreno's sociometric tools, such as the sociogram, are research instruments used in the study of communication dynamics in groups. Even studies of the *rhetoric of goodbye* as efforts to discover how people terminate their encounters provide knowledge of the complex communication process.

The second way to improve our communication is to become more *aware of self*, of our intrapsychic environment, which harbors our needs, values, biases, and prejudices. Socrates gave good counsel when he said, "Know thyself." Few of us can say that we truly know self. What we do know about ourselves is generally very superficial and often inconsequential compared with what remains hidden. As the expression states, we need to "ladle from the bottom," reach deep down where the rich substance of *you* resides, and explore the needs, biases, and value system that have become the basis for our communication behavior. More will be said about the intrapersonal aspect of our communication system in the following chapter. We need to ask how and why we behave as we do; what needs, feelings, and thoughts are being expressed by certain utterances and actions. Once understood, some behavior may need to be changed.

It is important for each of us to search out the answers to the question "Who am I?" Our self-image is important to us personally and professionally and affects our intrapersonal and interpersonal communication. All communication begins with feelings about self and then involves feelings and philosophy about others. What assumptions do we have about ourself as a person and as a communicator? We must look at our own self-image because that determines how we present ourselves to others, how others perceive us, and how they respond to our messages. The false fronts may fool us but also hide our true self from others.

Much of our communication behavior functions outside our awareness. Through reflection and questioning, we can get in touch with our true feelings. The world is a ready-made laboratory for daily study of self and behavior. We can and must learn about our behavior through feedback from others.

We all have a cache of habits and routines that affect our behavior. Prather writes: "In order to break with a habit I will first have to become aware of how I usually act. I will have to see how I do it before I can undo it. At the time, I am not aware of how I shut down my attention or hold back my warmth."[11] Awareness of one's behavior is required before under-

---

[11]Hugh Prather, *I Touch the Earth, the Earth Touches Me*, Doubleday & Co., Garden City, N.Y., 1972, unpaged.

standing of it can occur, and both are essential to improving our communication behavior.

The third general way to improve our communication relates to our interpersonal communication and requires that we become more *sensitive to others*. It is not enough to verbally acknowledge individual differences in communication behavior. We must be continuously sensitive to these differences and adjust our symbols and stimuli to accommodate them. We do little in our educational programs to help students learn how to improve their perceptual acuity, yet it is so essential to all interpersonal activities of life. No two people see alike, for no two have the same life experiences, which serve as their frame of reference or base of operation. We must learn to "walk in the other fellow's shoes" and to "see the world through his eyes."

Experiential learning not only helps us to improve our understanding of the communication process per se but also is useful as a means for gaining understanding about self and sensitivity toward others. Entire books are devoted to communication games and exercises. The number of personal growth experience workshops and encounter group activities is legion.

OVERVIEW OF REMAINDER OF THE BOOK

The intent of this book is to help the reader gain a comprehensive picture of the human communication process as it operates in our personal and professional lives. It is indeed frustrating to find that the study of human communication, which so deeply touches the lives of each of us, has received so little attention at all levels of our educational system. In most curricula in the health fields, there is a dearth of discrete courses focusing on communication theories and methodologies.

The content of this book has global application. Nothing relating to the human communication process per se is particularly unique to any person or professional group. Numerous examples will be cited and analogies made in an effort to aid the reader in more clearly understanding and applying the general concepts. The examples and applications are directed toward communication as it relates to the nursing profession. The aspects of the communication process which have been touched on in this introductory chapter will be elaborated upon throughout the book.

Part I includes a model of human communication, an intrapersonal model. This model also serves as the basis for our interpersonal communication with the addition of other relevant variables that impinge upon communication in dyads and groups. A chapter is devoted to the all-important and unique characteristic of man as a symbolizing animal. A separate chapter is devoted to the temporal and spatial dimensions of communication. Frequently time and space are relegated to a mere mention under the rubric "nonverbal communication." The communication contract that is a part of all communication exchange is discussed under a separate chapter heading. A chapter is devoted to dysfunctional communication; it should shed light on some of our common communication problems and potential barriers to effective communication. A generous portion of the chapter focuses on suggested methods for bridging the barriers. Principles of general semantics provide one means of preventing as well as correcting some of our semantic ills.

Presented in Part II is a pragmatic approach, an application of principles and concepts presented in Part I to a number of selected functional areas of nursing practice, education, and administration. The functional areas selected for presentation are in no way to be construed as the most important functions of nursing, nor are they all-inclusive. Those areas selected merely reflect the bias of the author and the need to limit the scope of this undertaking. They include the nursing process, the nurse-client relationship, the teaching-learning process, management, and change. Some, if not all, of those selected should be of concern to all students, clinicians, nursing administrators, and educators. A few of the most appropriate communication concepts are discussed in detail under each functional area.

The multitude of variables to be considered and the complexity with which they interact with one another, together with the inherent uncertainty of attaining effective communication, should not be viewed as meaning that the task is unpleasant or impossible. It is a worthwhile challenge that pays high rewards. The material presented is directed toward the ultimate goal of helping the nurse, irrespective of position or field of employment, become a more effective communicator and thereby more responsive to the health care needs of our society.

SUGGESTED BIBLIOGRAPHY

Beer, Stafford: *Cybernetics and Management*, John Wiley & Sons, New York, 1959 (3rd printing, 1967).

Brooks, William D.: *Speech Communication*, Wm. C. Brown Co., Publishers, Dubuque, Iowa, 1971.

Dance, Frank E. X. (ed.): *Human Communication Theory: Original Essays*, Holt, Rinehart and Winston, New York, 1967.

Haley, Jay (ed.): *Changing Families: A Family Therapy Reader*, Grune & Stratton, New York, 1971.

Kibler, Robert J. and Larry L. Barker (eds.): *Conceptual Frontiers in Speech-Communication: Report of the New Orleans Conference on Research and Instructional Development*, Speech Association of America, New York, 1969.

Korzybski, Alfred: *Manhood of Humanity*, 2d ed., The International Non-Aristotelian Library Publishing Co., Lakeville, Conn., 1950.

Krupar, Karen R.: *Communication Games*, Free Press, New York, 1973.

Lewin, Kurt: *Field Theory in Social Science: Selected Theoretical Papers*, Harper & Row, Publishers, New York, 1951.

McCroskey, James C.: *An Introduction to Rhetorical Communication*, 2d ed., Prentice-Hall, Englewood Cliff, N.J., 1972.

Miller, George A. (ed.): *Communication, Language, and Meaning: Psychological Perspectives*, Basic Books, New York, 1973.

Murray, Elwood, Gerald M. Phillips, and J. David Truby: *Speech: Science-Art*, The Bobbs-Merrill Co., Indianapolis, Ind., 1969.

Smith, Alfred G. (ed.): *Communication and Culture*, Holt, Rinehart and Winston, New York, 1966.

Wiener, Norbert.: *The Human Use of Human Beings*, Houghton Mifflin, Boston, 1950.

Chapter 2

An Intrapersonal Human Communication Model

Every man is a volume if you know how to read him.

Channing

Human communication is a relatively new field of study. While a multitude of concepts and theories abound, scientific testing of them is only in the embryonic stage. In fact, specialists in speech communication have been spending time trying to identify the realistic parameters of research in the field. Model building, which often accompanies theoretical development, has been used as an aid in conceptualizing and understanding the communication phenomenon.

MODELS AND THEIR USES

A *model* is a pictorial means of representing a theory or a way of viewing and explaining a process. Models, like the theories they represent, are hypothetical and subjective. They generally consist of a line drawing or a diagram of a series of events or pheonomena showing their relationship to one another. Models have been found useful as a means of organizing constructs as well as isolating and showing the functional relationships of elements in a complex system. As a copy or representation of the actual process as perceived, a model can serve as a point of reference for discussion and as a conceptual device to aid us to visualize and thereby explain, explore, and study a process. Voids and faulty conceptualization often become evident to the theorist through model building and may guide him in reexamining his original thinking.

While compactness and simplicity characterize models and the reason for using them, there is a tendency to *oversimplify* a complex process and thereby distort it. There are limits to what can be included in a model and how complex interactions can be portrayed in diagram form. Frequently, as with a model of human communication, one is limited by the black Box phenomenon: the unknowns and missing parts. Predictability is a characteristic quality of most models, especially in the physical sciences, where cause-and-effect relationships often can be established.

SOME MODELS OF HUMAN COMMUNICATION

There is no *one* accepted theory or model of human communication. Most of the model building relating to human communication appeared just prior to and during the 1950s. The development of information theory began with Wiener,[1] the mathematician who introduced the concept of *control* and regulation of machines and of communication of information.

The Shannon-Weaver communication model (Figure 2-1) is a classic in the field and has served as the basis for a wide assortment of modified versions. The simple block diagram reduces the complex process to a few essential elements. The key parameters of the communication system are modeled as information source, transmitter, channel, noise source, receiver, and message destination. The information source and message destination are generally the individuals involved in the communication process and are often referred to as the *encoder* (sender) and *decoder* (receiver) respectively. Noise is incorporated into the model as an interfering signal.

The Berlo SMCR model[2] includes the basic components of source, message, channel, and receiver but adds some of the human variables that affect the processing of messages. Included are such factors as communication skills, attitudes, knowledge, and social and cultural variables.

[1]Norbert Wiener, *Cybernetics,* John Wiley & Sons, New York, 1948.
[2]David K. Berlo, *The Process of Communication: An Introduction to Theory and Practice,* Holt, Rinehart & Winston, New York, 1960, p. 72.

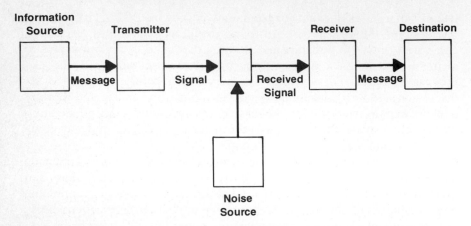

Figure 2-1 Shannon-Weaver communication model. *(Claude E. Shannon and Warren Weaver, The Mathematical Theory of Communication, University of Illinois Press, Urbana, Ill., 1949, p. 98. Reprinted by permission of publisher.)*

Most of the communication models that have been developed are *interpersonal* models. To this author, these models fail to do justice to the complex human processing of information which lies at the core of human communication. These models frequently are mathematical or represent computer operations, and as has already been stated, are too mechanistic, deterministic, and simplistic to represent the human data processing system. While data processing performed by humans does bear *some* similarity to characteristics of data processing by machines, many human qualities are antithetical, rendering the mathematical models both inadequate and inaccurate. While there is some patterning to human data processing, there is also much caprice within the system.

No useful purpose can be served by either describing or belaboring the inadequacies of models that have already been developed. The reader is encouraged to review theories and models in more detail as they appear in many of the speech communication texts.

AN INTRAPERSONAL COMMUNICATION MODEL

If the communication process were as simple as many of the theories and models would lead one to believe, we would not experience the communication problems we do today. Such is not the case, however, for when the human element is given its due respect and logical place at the core of the process, the answer to why communication difficulties are so prevalent becomes readily apparent.

The intrapersonal communication model that is presented here and the theory behind it represent the author's attempt to capture and explain the true essence of man as data gatherer, generator, processor, and transformer. The task is not an easy one, for we have no *direct* way of knowing what actually goes on as humans use messages to generate and transmit meaning. Our knowledge must come mainly from the inferences we draw from overt responses. This indirect source of information obviously leaves us with many questions not only about the intended message itself but also about the actual patterning of events in the process. In this model, such constructs as sensation, perception, cognition, symbolization, memory, and overt behavior are organized into a theoretical structure to help visualize and improve our understanding and, to a degree, predict and control human communication behavior. Our understanding of the cognitive process remains limited even though its importance to communication activities is without question. Hidden in man's inner world is the complex functioning and some of the mystery of how he perceives and sends messages and generates meaning.

In an effort to conceptualize the sequence of events—how messages take on meaning and eventuate in a response—we must grasp some notion of the interface between an individual's *external* and *internal* environments. Information exists only as a result of a relationship between external (and at times internal) stimuli and one's internal state. It is not so much a matter of what happens in the external environment per se—the message stimulus—but how a person perceives those events that will determine meaning and a response. It is the biased view of this author that in the past, too much importance has erroneously been placed on the stimulus or message.

The communication process is deeply rooted in one's personality, in the internal state of the individuals involved. An objective view of the world is impossible. Only through contact with others, through socialization, can we attempt to verify "our" reality, but even then we must be content to learn only how close or distant we are to one another in our sensory and perceptual fields. In fact we do not really know that the color we label "bright red" is anywhere near the shade sensed and perceived by another individual. To the individual who is color blind, the colors are real to him. It may take years before he realizes, through discourse with others, that he has a sensory defect. Many of our communication problems can be traced to the common but false assumption that there is *one* real world and that is the one *we* view.

We create a world that will suit our purpose and as the constraints, particularly internal ones, dictate. We are continuously at work, mostly at an unconscious level, preparing our internal system for the production of meaning. We literally invent ourselves, our environment, and the people in it. The *unique* world that is of our own creation is the result of our unique sensory, perceptual, and symbolic processing of stimuli. While few would dispute the concept of individual differences, we often behave and communicate as though each of us had identical sensory and cognitive experiences. Henry David Thoreau said: "If a man does not keep pace with his companions, perhaps it is because he hears a different drummer. Let him step to the music which he hears, however measured or far away." We must not only respect this individuality but also be continuously aware of it as we attempt to improve our understanding of and skill in communicating with self and others.

There is a story of three baseball umpires, each of whom was asked how he distinguished a ball from a strike. Each of their responses conveys a communication principle. The first umpire said, "There are balls and there are strikes and I calls them *as I see them*." His statement relates to the fact that each person can describe the event only as gathered through his unique sensory and perceptual fields. The second umpire said, "There are balls and there are strikes and I calls them *as they is*." His response exemplifies the common misconception that we all perceive alike. The third umpire exclaimed, "There are balls and there are strikes but they *ain't nothing* until I calls them." His answer speaks to the point that there may be stimuli but they are without meaning, they are nothing, until they are perceived and processed. Again, there is no reality, no world out there except as each individual constructs it. One is reminded of the eternal question "If a tree falls in the forest and no one is there, does it make a noise?" The intrapersonal communication model may help us glean some new insights or at least develop some new ways to consider the answer to that question.

The intrapersonal model presented in Figure 2-2 has been developed and will be used as a source of reference for further content presented throughout this book. While much of our concern will center around *inter*personal communication activities in dyadic, intragroup, intergroup, and multigroup personal and professional settings, the thesis behind employing an *intra*personal model to explain all human communication processes is the recognition that the intrapersonal, or internal, processing of messages is the core of all interpersonal communication as well. The intrapersonal model of person A placed in juxtaposition with the intrapersonal model of person B represents the *interpersonal* communication activities in that dyad, as shown in Figure 2-3. The response, for example, a word symbol uttered by person A, becomes the external stimulus for person B, with the potential of being sensed and perceived and producing meaning and a response.

As the model is studied, the reader is reminded of the dilemma that is inherent in model building, which requires a choice between using a simple linear model for greater understanding and clarity or a complex, multidimensional model that may more accurately reflect the process but be as difficult to interpret as to construct. In arriving at somewhat of a com-

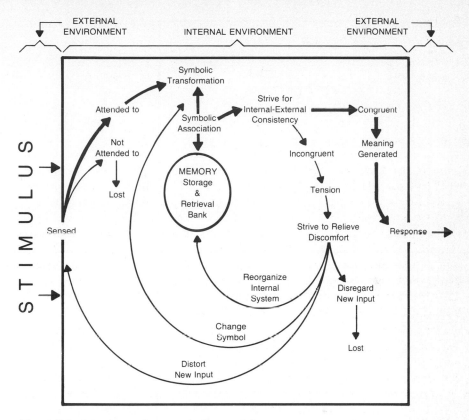

Figure 2-2 Intrapersonal communication model.

promise, the reader is asked to keep a number of factors in mind. There actually is no discrete, stepwise sequence of events, as might be erroneously inferred from the model. Various activities, particularly in the perceptual phase of the communication process, go on simultaneously, and there is interplay in both directions as symbolic transformation and symbolic association are tested with stored data. At any stage in the process, the transformed stimulus may be disregarded or distorted or the symbolic form modified. As is true of any theory, any model may indeed generate more questions than answers.

The human data processing system, from the point of sensation of stimuli to overt behavior or response, involves our *sense organs, spinal cord and its extensions,* and *brain.* The total process takes place at various levels of consciousness. Our sense organs pick up certain external (and internal) stimuli through sight, sound, taste, touch, smell, and temperature sensation. The nervous system functions to process these perceived stimuli into symbolic form and associate, or check them out, with the

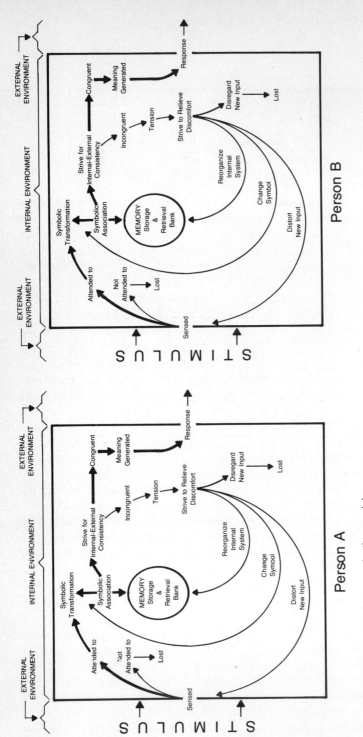

Figure 2-3 Interpersonal communication model.

symbolic categories that have been stored in memory. The brain functions as a transformer as well as a transmitter of messages. The brain has its own laws that dictate if and how new symbolic inputs will be processed. Our nervous system serves as the link between the data perceived and the stored symbolic past. As shown in the model (Figure 2-2), we have patterns in our brains and we organize, filter, and select stimuli as we strive for a degree of consistency between internal and external inputs.

Sensation

To live in the world, we must receive information from that world. The sense organs, or *receptors*, initiate the process of information gathering that helps ensure our survival. A constant stream of stimuli bombards the nerve endings of our sense organs every minute of our lives. Studies have revealed that outside stimuli impinge upon our internal environment even during sleep. Stimuli may be verbal or nonverbal, animate or inanimate. These stimuli are disorganized and unprocessed data primarily from our external environment which have the *potential* of being sensed and initiating the production of meaning. Some stimuli will be tended to, and others will be ignored. Communication cannot take place, of course, if the stimulus is ignored. The sensory phase is primarily a physical process of stimulation of the nerve endings and is largely unconscious. For example, we sense the pressure of a chair against our body *only* when we attend to it and thereby bring it into the consciousness of our perception.

While most stimuli, or messages, originate from our external environment, there are also stimuli that are internally generated. Internal stimuli might include our phobias and our organ responses to hunger, thirst, pain, fatigue, and the like. For example, external stimuli sensed by person A might be a statement from person B, "It's time for lunch"; seeing or smelling food on the table; observing that the hands of a clock are on 12 o'clock; or hearing the clock strike 12 at midday. A single internal stimulus might be a felt hunger pain. It is conceivable that all these stimuli might be present simultaneously and produce a series of messages (stimuli) which would reinforce one another and increase the chances of being sensed by person A. The clock designating 12 noon probably would not be sensed or perceived as meaning "time for lunch." if that was not the individual's usual time for lunch.

Some of our internal and external stimuli may not be sensed because of physical or emotional defects. Deaf and/or blind individuals may feel isolated from the world, which has so many stimuli that must be sensed by auditory and visual receptors. Our imagination may run wild and distort our sensual experience; yet we need sensory inputs to communicate and to survive.

Some of our sense organs have greater acuity and are better developed for picking up stimuli than others are. When one sense organ is impaired, another may serve a collateral function and increase its receptivity to stimuli. Helen Keller, who could neither see nor hear, developed a keen sense of touch. A dog's sense of smell is far more developed than that of humans. We cannot smell a pheasant ahead of us in a field, but a hunting dog picks up the scent of the bird 20 or 50 feet ahead, follows the bird, and flushes it from the brush. The hunter must wait for his auditory and visual sense organs to locate the bird before he can make the kill. It has been speculated that our abundant use of deodorants and perfumes has further reduced man's potential to communicate through his sense of smell.

Interesting comparisons have been made between the sensory abilities of man and those of animals. For example, a frog's eye does not see a fly as we see it, with all of its parts. In fact, a frog cannot spot a fly unless it moves. Studies have shown that a frog in a cage with freshly killed insects will actually starve to death.

Fear and threat can modify our sensory acuity. The mother hears even the soft respirations and slightest noise of the sick child in an adjoining room. The frightened client becomes more sensitive to the noise on the hospital unit.

Stimulus overload can be as emotionally and physically unhealthy as sensory deprivation. Confusion and a state of constant fatigue might be the dubious reward for sensing and attending to the plethora of stimuli that tickle our senses. We might be subject to psychoses through the recycling of our internal inputs, our dreams and fantasies.

Perception

Not everything that has been sensed will be attended to and perceived, but nothing can be perceived until it first has been sensed. Perception is undoubtedly the most important as well as the most complex aspect of human behavior. Unsuccessful efforts have been made to study and simulate the complex perceptual and cognitive processes of man through computer science. Freudian psychology has offered some explanation of the role of unconscious motivation in the selection and rejection of stimuli. Theories on the effects of early childhood experiences on our selective process have been advanced by Pavlovian psychologists. Some studies have been directed toward identifying perceptual differences between the sexes. For example, the findings from one such study revealed that women of all ages are visually more aware of their surroundings than men are. The theories of perception are unending, yet much of it remains a mystery as well as a marvel.

Perception takes place primarily at the conscious level, and the brain is the seat of all perception. It is at the perceptual level that meaning is generated through the symbolic process. As displayed in the model, the perceptual phase includes *attending to* what has been sensed, giving *order and structure* to the raw sensed data through *symbolic transformation*, and making *associations* between the new inputs and symbolic categories of past events that are stored and retrieved from *memory*. Perception involves the selection, organization, and interpretation of specific stimuli that have been sensed. Perception is impossible if either the sensory or the symbolic process does not function.

The possibility that the sensed data will be attended to and thereby the perceptual phase of the communication process will begin depends upon the *perceived utility value* or need that the individual has for the information *at that particular time*. For example, we may perceive a bowl of fruit on the table before we eat, but it might never reach perceptual awareness after we have satisfied our hunger. We may drive down the same street day after day and never notice the gasoline station on the corner until we have an urgent need to fill our gas tank. Likewise, an article on breast cancer may become evident to us only after we discover a suspicious breast lesion. This discriminating activity may offer some explanation for what otherwise might be interpreted as inconsistent behavior on the part of another individual. Man actually is rational, and his behavior and reality make sense *to him*.

Powerful internal directives control if and how new inputs will be assimilated. If a sensed stimulus is perceived as a threat to our internal environment, we may "narrow our vision" and ignore it. As we make our own reality, we reject, distort, and modify sensed data to suit our fancy.

Another principle that operates as we perceive sensed data is our ability to take in and attend to *only one thing at a time*. When we ride in a taxi and are concerned with the cost of the trip, the meter blocks our view of the beautiful flower garden along the way. If we have two earphones in place and a different message is sent into each, we ignore one and attend to the other if appropriate.

In our perception, we experience distortions in the form of illusions and hallucinations. The angle at which we approach a stimulus dictates our sensory and perceptual response. How many golfers walk down the fairway with their eyes on their round, white golf ball, only to find as they get closer to it that it has become a rectangular, white piece of paper? The fact that we often find someone else's lost golf ball but not our own may also be explained in terms of our sensory and perceptual functions. Have you ever looked at the world from the physical plane of a child? A child's sense of perspective and spatial relationships is quite different from that of an adult. One reason the same event may be viewed differently by an adult and a child is that each is physically viewing his world from a different spatial level or plane.

Bringing order and structure to our unprocessed sensory experiences occurs at the perception stage, when we deal with *relationships* and *symbolic form*. Symbols are created from human thought and result from a synthesis of the sensed stimulus with the inner world. Stimuli furnished through the senses are constantly being transformed into symbols that serve as our coding system. Symbols are representations of objects, events, and people; they stand for something or someone. Words are our most commonly used symbols. Symbols are learned culturally or through social convention. All human behavior involves man's symbolic process. The symbol-generating capacity is a uniquely human function.

After our incoming perceptions have undergone symbolic transformation, they are categorized in relation to our unique internal program, which has been patterned from a lifetime of experiences and stored for retrieval from our memory bank. The sensed data must be placed in some context, in some relationship and symbolic association with the memory bank, for them to be of any use. The more experiences one has stored in one's memory and available for retrieval, the greater the capacity one has for making subtle but useful symbolic associations. For example, the word "chair" may only represent "something to sit on" to many individuals. However, for others, their stored information is joined with existing needs, and other associations may be made. For example, a "chair" might represent "firewood" to an individual who is freezing to death in a cabin, a "crutch" to one who needs support to keep from bearing weight on an injured foot, or a "ladder" to one who needs to extend his reaching capability. A "chair" may be of no value and may not enter one's perceptual awareness except as the stimulus (chair) symbolically represents something needed at that time.

Symbolization, the capacity to develop a system of meaningful symbols, is one of man's unique communication abilities. Through the use of symbols, man has yet another unique ability, that of *binding time*. We can preserve and recall the past as we relate symbols to experiences and events retrieved from our storage bank (memory) and thereby generate meaning. The brain is our filing cabinet, filled with stored symbols. There is no agreement on how memory functions, but we do know that it is vitally important to the communication system of man. The quality of the communication behavior of lower animals is inferior to that of man because they lack the ability to symbolize and time-bind.

Some experiences may never be stored in memory. Others may be stored but repressed and inaccessible except as revealed through dreams and psychotherapy. Experiences may be more easily recalled if they are recent, repeated, or particularly significant to us. Events are generally more strongly fixed in memory if they have been experiences of youth and more vivid in recall if they result from crisis situations.

Just as DNA is the genetic substance that gives us *our* uniqueness, so our *internal frame of reference* determines the unique message meaning that is generated through our perceptual field. A few examples of how we perceive from our own frame of reference might help clarify and reinforce this important concept.

Three men were standing on the southern rim of the Grand Canyon, looking down into the massive canyon below. One was a priest, another an artist, and the third a cowboy. The priest conveyed his perception and meaning when he said, "What a wonderful creation of God." The artist reflected, "What a beautiful picture to paint." The cowboy exclaimed, "What a hell of a place to lose a cow!" Each individual was seemingly exposed to the same external visual stimulus but generated very different meaning based on a unique frame of reference.

Another illustration of unique and private perceptions is revealed from the comments of five small children when they were shown a picture of the Mona Lisa and were asked by their teacher, "Why is she smiling?" Something about each child's frame of reference is evident from their responses:

She backed the car out without scraping it.

Her husband was drying dishes, and she had nothing to do.

They have a nice family and a good baby.

She went to the race track and won $5000.

She was cold, and someone turned on the heat.

Our behavior as a reflection of the reality we create may make sense to us but seem irrational to someone else. A boy was hunting rabbits with his father, and the father shot a rabbit. He cut off one foot of the rabbit, gave it to the boy, and said, "Here, son, this is for you for good luck." Obviously not knowing of the conventional association between a rabbit's foot and good luck, the boy said, "Gee, Dad, the rabbit had four of them and look what happened to him!"

Perceptual bias was further evident from the conversation between a lawyer and a plumber. The lawyer, who perceived the job of a plumber as rather demeaning work, said to the plumber, "I can't see how you can gain much satisfaction from *that* kind of work." "Oh, but you are wrong," said the plumber. "It is very satisfying and rewarding work, for every time I repair a faucet and turn on the water, I am releasing water from the mountains 90 miles away." It is all in how we change sensed stimuli into symbols and produce meaning. Everything has beauty but not everyone sees it, for beauty is in the eye of the beholder.

Most of our ineffective interpersonal communication can be attributed to these unique perceptions that generate very different meanings. However, there are also benefits to be gained from these diverse ways of viewing our world. As Barnlund said: "It is these differences in perception that make communication inevitable. If men saw the same facts in the same way, there would be no reason to talk at all. . . . There would be no experiences to share, no conflicts to negotiate."[3] It would indeed be a dull and lonely world!

Much of our data processing behavior is unconsciously geared toward maintaining a degree of harmony between our external and internal environments. To survive psychologically, we must perceive our reality as reasonably constant and stable. In fact, our communication behavior is more a reflection of these internal constraints, as stated previously, than of the external stimulus. We strive to avoid dissonance as the ordered and symbolic perceptions come in contact with our inner laws.

We would be remiss in our discussion of perception and man's need for order, structure, and unity if we did not address the concepts of *determinism* and *free will*. What kinds of constraints are present in one's internal environment which to a varying degree determine or limit the inputs that can be assimilated? How free are individuals to take in new inputs, especially when they are incongruent with those stored and retrieved from memory? Is there a uniqueness to the way individuals respond to this *internal noise* of dissonance which may force them to reject, distort, and modify data? We have a tenacious past. In fact, the past is *not* past, for it molds our personality and becomes the fabric of our present and future communication behavior.

Our perceptual selectivity or discrimination reduces our need to cope with discrepant information; yet opposing perceptions do help to stimulate thought. As shown in the intrapersonal model (Figure 2-2), we reject and modify information as we attempt to make it congruent with our symbolic past. At times we may even reorganize our internal storage program or reorder and change the input symbols. Royce[4] referred to man as "encapsulated" and imprisoned by his own inner constraints, his biases, prejudices, stereotypes, and value system. Our should and should not system dictates our behavior.

Many questions remain, such as: To what degree can each of us tolerate the tensions and discomfort produced by inconsistencies? What price is each of us willing to pay to change, and what rewards can we

[3]Dean C. Barnlund, "Communication: The Context of Change," in Carl E. Larson and Frank E. X. Dance (eds.), *Perspectives on Communication,* Speech Communication Center, University of Wisconsin, Milwaukee, 1968, p. 26.
[4]Joseph R. Royce, *The Encapsulated Man,* D. Van Nostrand Co., Princeton, N.J., 1964.

expect? What are the payoffs for making changes in the internal system? Will they compensate for the discomfort and tension experienced in the process of resolving the incongruities?

At this point it seems appropriate to add to our knowledge about the communication process by reviewing a few of the more well-known theories relating to our efforts to maintain internal/external harmony. We are certain that people are not like clay, to be easily molded by new external inputs. In fact, most individuals are more like cement, all mixed up and permanently set!

The theory of *self-consistency* as developed by Lecky[5] claims that everyone must be true to himself and must do so by reducing intrapersonal conflict or inconsistencies within the system itself. A person can move in only one direction at a time and likewise can believe only one thing at a time. The object of integrative forces within the individual is to preserve unity and prevent the tension and discomfort experienced when contradictions exist.

According to Lecky there is *psychic determinism*, in which each event is determined by what precedes it. Ideas that are consistent with the stored past tend to be assimilated, while those that are inconsistent tend to be rejected. Forgetting, as viewed by Lecky, is not accidental but actually planned. If the prize is big enough, one might rearrange and change his inner self.

Festinger's theory of *cognitive dissonance* is similar to Lecky's self-consistency theory. When an individual is confronted with information contrary to his own, he experiences dissonance and engages in activities to reduce the discomfort.[6] Individuals maintain control by dictating what can enter the system. Persons experience tension if forced to act in a manner contrary to their inner program. Incongruent beliefs and attitudes cannot be held simultaneously. In other words, we strive "not to rock the boat." Festinger contends that the relevancy and importance of the data to the individual and the credibility attached to the person who might be voicing the dissonant data affect what may be taken into the system.

Wiener's major contribution to information theory was the concept of *homeostasis*.[7] He proposed that we use *negative feedback* to correct discrepancies between desired and observed data. When there is deviation from the desired state, efforts are made to correct for these disturbances.

The work of Harvey focused upon attempting to explain why some

[5] Prescott Lecky, *Self-Consistency: A Theory of Personality*, The Shoe String Press, Hamden, Conn., 1961.
[6] Leon Festinger, *A Theory of Cognitive Dissonance*, Row, Peterson and Co., New York, 1957.
[7] Wiener, *Cybernetics*.

individuals have greater tolerance for dissonance than others and have more open internal systems.[8] He developed an instrument (This I Believe Test) to measure the conceptual systems, or levels of *concreteness-abstractness*, of people. He identified four categories of people, from System I concrete to System IV abstract. Harvey theorized that each of us has a belief or value system that serves as a set of predispositions for taking in and interpreting stimuli. Some individuals tolerate dissonance more than others do.

Harvey and his associates have conducted numerous related studies over the past decade and a half. They have categorized and characterized individuals who fall into each of the four conceptual systems. They found that the most System I concrete individuals are very intolerant of ambiguity and make up their minds more completely based on little information.[9] System IV abstract individuals, who unfortunately are least in number of those studied, are more open-minded, flexible, adaptable, and creative. The conceptual system of the adults studied was found to be associated with characteristics of their child-parent relationships.

Research findings provide rather convincing evidence to support, at least to some extent, a deterministic philosophy of the human processing of information. Much of our observed behavior is indicative of the inherent effort made to avoid change and maintain internal-external harmony. Knowing about the complex communication process will help us, but what may be even more beneficial is to know more about the individual with whom we are attempting to develop effective communication. If we knew, for example, that the individual was a System IV abstract person, we might be able to predict that we could exert influence on him because his system would be open to change. Obviously there is a degree of free will, of power to choose without restraints, in most if not all of us. Yet we find it hard to overcome the internal environment we build for ourselves.

SUGGESTED BIBLIOGRAPHY

Berlo, David K.: *The Process of Communication: An Introduction to Theory and Practice*, Holt, Rinehart & Winston, Inc., New York, 1960.
Brooks, William D.: *Speech Communication*, Wm. C. Brown Co., Publishers, Dubuque, Iowa, 1971.
Budd, Richard W. and Brent D. Ruben: *Approaches to Human Communication*, Spartan Books, New York, 1972.

[8]O. J. Harvey, D. E. Hunt, and H. M. Schroder, *Conceptual Systems and Personality Organization*, John Wiley & Sons, New York, 1961.
[9]Alma Grabow Miller and O. J. Harvey, "Effects of Concreteness-Abstractness and Anxiety on Intellectual and Motor Performance," *Journal of Consulting and Clinical Psychology*, **40**(3):444–451, 1973.

Cherry, Colin: *On Human Communication*, John Wiley & Sons, New York, 1957.
———— (ed.): *Pragmatic Aspects of Human Communication,* D. Reidel Publishing
    Co., Boston, 1974.
Harvey, O.J. (ed.): *Motivation and Social Interaction: Cognitive Determinants*,
    The Ronald Press Co., New York, 1963.
Newcomb, Theodore M.: "An Approach to the Study of Communicative Acts,"
    Psychological Review, **60:**393–404, November 1953.
Reitman, Walter R.: *Cognition and Thought: An Information-Processing Ap-
    proach*, John Wiley & Sons, New York, 1965.
Shannon, Claude E. and Warren Weaver: *The Mathematical Theory of Communi-
    cation*, University of Illinois Press, Urbana, Ill., 1949.
Ware, Robert and O. J. Harvey: "A Cognitive Determinant of Impression Forma-
    tion," *Journal of Personality and Social Psychology*, **5**(1):38–44, 1967.
Wiener, Norbert: *The Human Use of Human Beings*, 2d ed., Doubleday & Co.,
    Garden City, N.Y., 1954.

Chapter 3

Our Symbolic World

Sometimes when I consider what tremendous consequences come from little things—a chance word, a tap on the shoulder, or a penny dropped on a news-stand,—
I am tempted to think—there are no "little things."

Bruce Barton

We make our own reality, and it is a world of symbols. Meaning, the essence of human communication, is generated from stimuli through the symbolic process. Because of the importance symbols play in the communication process, it seemed appropriate to devote a chapter to a discussion of the galaxy of symbols we create, manipulate, and use during our lifetime.

Man constantly engages in symbolic thought and expression, reflects on objects and events, and relates to others through a unique coding system. Our entire existence revolves around changing stimuli into symbols that have meaning to us. While words are our most commonly used symbols, there are equally important nonverbal symbols, such as gestures and body movement. Through our use of symbols we can express virtually every experience and thought.

SYMBOLS

Symbols are anything that take the place of, stand for, or refer to something or someone. It is obvious that we cannot carry around people, objects, and events to point to as we attempt to convey messages to others; so our code becomes a handy replacement. Messages are transmitted in symbolic form. The symbols have the potential to take on meaning through the perceptual process, as diagramed in the intrapersonal communication model presented in the previous chapter.

Symbols are man-made, arbitrary, and subject to continual revision. Anything that can be produced by one man can be distorted and destroyed by another; that holds true for creating symbols. Man the symbol maker not only attaches his unique meaning to symbols but also develops new symbols to represent objects or individuals that may have traditionally been identified by other symbols. For example, there is nothing to keep us from using the word symbol "casing" instead of "skin" as the referent for the outer layer of our body tissue.

The symbol is not the thing itself; it is only a code used in referring to the thing. Problems of semantics develop as we fool ourselves into thinking of and reacting to symbols as if they were the real thing. For example, by repeating the word symbols "lemon, lemon is sour, very, very sour," we may soon find ourself salivating as though we were actually sucking on a lemon. If we were handed a plate of food and someone labeled it "dog food," we would probably react to the label and refuse to eat it. Abuse of the symbolic process may result in serious psychological problems. In fact, a characteristic of many individuals suffering mental illness is the ingenious way in which they manipulate word symbols.

We evaluate and create symbols and then assign meaning in terms of their use to us. A symbol may induce meaning in one context but have no meaning in another. The setting and occasion influence the generation of meaning. For example, "ice skates" would probably be meaningless to a child living on a tropical island, or at least would not have the same meaning as it would for a child living in the midwestern United States. For a drunk, a lamppost may have meaning as a source of support but not as a source of illumination. Symbols cannot be studied or understood in isolation. They take on meaning only as they appear in some context. Cultural patterning also affects symbolic meaning.

It is fortunate that although individuals engage in unique symbolic processing of stimuli, through tradition and universal usage many symbols take on rather consistent meaning. If this were not the case, our ability to function as a civilized society would be in jeopardy. Symbols must generate some universally accepted meaning between and among individuals for effective communication to occur.

The communication system of plants and animals is equally fascinating and complex, but differs from that of humans in the inability of these organisms to use verbal language. Animals use chemicals and glandular substances as well as specific movements, vocalizations, and color changes as they relate to one another. For example, the honeybee communicates by means of the direction and angle of its flight. This is referred to as the honeybee "waggle dance." The stare plays a key role in dominance relationships among rhesus monkeys. The stare is used as a display of aggression and hostility.

Birds reflect their hostility by ruffling their feathers and spreading their wings to give the illusion of bigness. Man exhibits similar behavior as he expands his chest in a gesture of strength, but his use of words as weapons cannot be overestimated. We can "put someone down" as quickly and as harshly with words as with a blow.

The choice of communication codes is limited to 10 to 37 for lower animals, compared with an infinite number for humans. Most of this human superiority as well as the problems in the field of communication relate to man's ability to symbolize, particularly to his use of verbal language. While the codes used by lower animals are stereotyped in meaning, uncertainty of meaning remains primarily a *human* communication problem.

VERBAL LANGUAGE

Our reality is a Niagara of symbols of many types. Johnson appropriately referred to symbols as "legal tender" for the exchange of information.[1] Spoken and written words are the most commonly used human symbols.

One of our problems with words is that individuals tend to operate on the false premise that a specific word automatically conveys a particular meaning to everyone. The meaning is not in the word symbol, but in the people who use the word. Having one world with a single language would accomplish little, for we would remain far apart in terms of having *one* meaning. Hall made that fact abundantly clear when he said, "There is no underlying connection, no inherent and inescapable relationship between any linguistic form and what it signifies."[2]

Verbal language is man's most important tool. Daniel Webster conveyed the value he placed on his ability to speak when he said, "If all my talents and powers were to be taken from me by some inscrutable Provi-

[1]Wendell Johnson, *People in Quandaries: The Semantics of Personal Adjustment,* Harper & Row, Publishers, New York, 1946, p. 91.
[2]Robert A. Hall, Jr., *Linguistics and Your Language,* Doubleday and Co., Garden City, N.Y., 1950, p. 123.

dence, and I had my choice of keeping but one, I would unhesitantly ask to be allowed to keep the Power of Speaking, for through it, I would quickly recover all the rest."

We are truly living in an oral generation. The airways are filled with sounds perceived as word symbols. We develop the ability to speak from a cry to a call to a word to a phrase. Our language serves not only as an instrument to form and express thought but also as a way to prevent, confuse, and conceal thought. Only through the complexities of our language has telling lies become possible. Untruths or ill-spoken words can do more damage than physical violence. One is led to question the saying, "Sticks and stones may break my bones but words will never hurt me."

Our language consists of grunts and scribbles or, as Thorndike referred to words, "only puffs of air or streaks of ink."[3] By convention we scribble in certain ways to produce letters and then arrange the letters into words and the words into sentences in an effort to elicit meaning and a response in others. Words, like doodles, are arbitrary codes. Look at the two doodles in Figures 3-1 and 3-2; before reading the caption, decide what symbolic meaning each has for you. To what extent do the captions under Figures 3-1 and 3-2 change the meaning generated by the pictures themselves? The beautiful mountains we see in the distance take on added and new meaning once we see the word symbols on a sign that reads, "The Mountain of the Kissing Camels." Which of the two figures (Figure 3-3 or 3-4) of lines and scrawls is the "golooma" and which is the "takiti"? Most

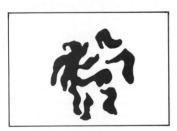

Figure 3-1 Doodles: An explosion in a spaghetti factory.

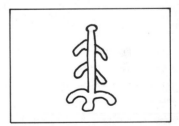

Figure 3-2 Doodles: A hall tree or coatrack for unwelcome guests.

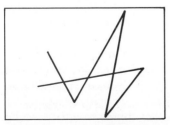

Figure 3-3 Lines and scrawls.

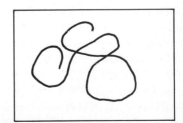

Figure 3-4 Lines and scrawls.

[3]Edward L. Thorndike, "The Psychology of Semantics," *The American Journal of Psychology,* 59:613, October 1946.

people assign the title "takiti" to Figure 3-3 and "golooma" to Figure 3-4. Contemplate and explore what was behind your symbolic associations and identification. Your answers may shed light on your unique symbolic processing system.

Meaning is not generated so much from single letter symbols as from the way in which the letters are arranged in relation to one another to form *words*. Look at the following six arrangements using the same three letters, A, T, and R, and become aware of your semantic reactions to each of the six words. Does each word generate some meaning for you through symbolic association?

ATR   RAT   TRA   RTA   TAR   ART

What effect do those words that may generate no meaning have on you? Do you find yourself trying to rearrange the letters so that they do have the potential to elicit meaning? Did you put the third word (TRA) into some kind of "tra la la" relationship? When a woman was asked if the RTA bothered her she said, "No, that is RITA." It was more than a coincidence, for her name happened to be Rita. Letters must be arranged in such a way that the word stands for something or someone and gives us a semantic reaction. If not, the word will result in *internal noise*, which can be frustrating and uncomfortable. Efforts will be made to disregard or modify the symbol. "The finest words in the world are only vain sounds, if you cannot comprehend them" (Anatole France).

Volume, tone of voice, and rate of speaking also affect message meaning. The last Senator Everett Dirksen of Illinois, the man with the deep voice, said, "The reason I keep my words soft, honeyed, and warm is because I never know when I may be called upon to eat them." A simple space or pause between letters in a word can make a dramatic difference in potential meaning: "I'm a person outstanding in my field" or "I'm a person out standing in my field." We use words in a certain context that allows us to be noncommital, for example, the response to the question "How do you like my new suit?" being "Well, it is different." What was commonly referred to in an address as Box Number has been renamed Drawer Number or even Container Number.

Semantic reactions are human responses of our nervous system to symbols, especially words, in relation to meaning. In the left column on page 45 are the more traditional words and labels, while in the right column are corresponding words that tend to conjure up a more positive image. Our aim in changing word symbols seems to be to get things to appear to be better than they are. For example, using the label "safety belt" could easily generate a semantic reaction of something *unsafe*, which was hardly the image the airline industry wanted to develop. Thus the label was changed to the healthier and more positive "seat belt." Words, like statistics, appear to lie, but it is really the people behind the statistical analysis and the words who manipulate data to suit their purpose.

Poverty	Low income
Slums or ghettos	Inner city
Prison	Correctional facility
Fired	Terminated or selected out
Late plane	Delayed departure
War Department	Department of Defense
Safety belt	Seat belt
Hospital	Body-repair shop
Partly cloudy	Mostly sunny
Disabled	Inconvenienced
Retirement	Readjustment
Garbage truck	Used-food purveyor
Dump	Sanitary fill
Bookie (in USA)	Turf accountant (in Ireland)
Earthquake	Real estate adjustment
Nude	Barefoot to the chin
Untidy house	Lived-in look
Salesperson	Personnel counselor
Janitor	Sanitary engineer

Meaning is not in the word but in people, yet as Locke said, "Men content themselves with the same words as other people use, as if the very sound necessarily carried the same meaning." There are even word symbols that are regionally unique. "Bubbler" is such a term; it is limited to the Midwest and is used to describe the drinking fountain on the corner of the city street or in a public building, which is kept "bubbling." "Guerney" is a term frequently employed on the West Coast to name something that may carry the label "stretcher" or "patient cart" in other sections of the country.

"Pig" had been the conventional label for the fat, short-legged barn-yard animal until the 1960s, when it became symbolic of law enforcement officers. It was used in an effort to denigrate the police, and it was used in that context for many years, until the police began referring to themselves as pigs. They attempted to and succeeded in using the symbol to generate a positive semantic reaction. They identified the word "pig" as standing for pride (P), integrity (I), and guts (G); and it immediately lost favor with the youth who had been using it in a derogatory fashion.

To coin new words is one thing, but to have them universally accepted into use is a more difficult problem. There are a number of classic examples of this problem in our health care system. For example, we continue our struggle to replace the term "medical care" with "health care" to more accurately reflect the multidisciplinary contributions to that care and foster a true health team approach. Adopting the term "medical treatment plan" to replace "doctor's orders," which implies a subservient role for the nurse as one under the doctor's command, will not be easy. We continue to hear the outdated term "bedside nurse" used when the concept on which it was based has changed dramatically over the years. Today most of our nursing care is provided in ambulatory health care settings that are generally void of beds rather than in the hospitals where, in years past, most clients were bedridden. Many nurses will recall the strong opposition voiced by physicians when we began using the term "nursing diagnosis." The doctors argued that "only doctors diagnose," and that the word "diagnose" was *their* word. It did not seem to matter that we were making *nursing*, not *medical*, diagnoses or that automobile mechanics and workers in other trades had been using the term "diagnose" for as long as one could remember. We do have territorial claims to words, ideas, and theories, which are protected by copyright laws, but there are limits.

A major linguistic change in the field of nursing has been the increasing use of the word "client" to replace the traditional label "patient." A brief description of the thinking behind it from one who has been actively involved in the change may be useful. Words are arbitrary, and they tend to become outdated as the events, people, and concepts they represent change. While engaged in a curriculum revision study in 1970, we found obvious dichotomies between the philosophy and objectives of the nursing program and the images that seemed to emerge when the term patient was used. The word patient quite logically in the past had come to represent an individual who was ill and confined to a hospital. However, that is not the case today, when most health care is provided in ambulatory care facilities and directed more toward prevention than toward care. Was an individual who came to the clinic for an annual physical examination to maintain good health to be labeled a patient? Over the years and before the Patients' Bill of Rights, the patient was only passively involved in care and truly was one who was worked *on* rather than worked *with*. Yet our objective was to foster a health team approach in which the individual seeking care would be an equal and active participant in the process. The word patient was too closely related to the word "patience." While patience was a useful virtue, as one was required to sustain long delays in seeing the doctor, that kind of image was not to be encouraged. Having individuals endure long waits for care should be neither an expected or an accepted policy in our health care delivery system. The "client" had become a familiar name in the field of counseling and pyschiatric nursing over the years and seemed to be a label with the potential of conveying the image that would be in concert with the philosophy and concepts of the program. A client is a consumer of services; one who is a peer, not a subordinate, as he seeks health care and advice. He is one who should actively participate in the planning, decision making, and implementation of the care he needs. The term client was in concert with the modern image of the health care consumer and therefore seemed appropriate as a replacement for patient on the health care scene.

Some of the traditionally accepted meanings elicited by specific words change with time. For example, prior to the Watergate era, "milk money" referred to the 5 or 10 cents given to a child to take to school to pay for milk. Since that time, milk money brings to mind the contributions made to the Nixon campaign fund by the American Dairy Association in exchange for special favors. Remember when "grass" referred to nothing but that green stuff on the ground around homes and parks? The image and potential meaning for the word "pot" seems to undergo changes with each new generation.

We do strange things with words. For example, how many of us say "That *sounds good*" as we read a recipe or a menu? We create pictures from words and virtually eat them. Some go "kitty corner" across the street; others think big and go "catty corner." We talk about "spitting *up*" something, yet how else can one spit but up? We "re"assure someone when chances are we never assured that person in the first place. We refer to "past" experience, yet when something has been experienced isn't it always past? Many of our savings and loan companies advertise that they give "free" gifts. That is redundant; for strictly speaking, if a gift is *not* free, it is not a gift. Have you ever wondered on what basis the weather forecaster chooses to report the weather as "partly cloudy" or "mostly sunny?"

Many words are popularized during a specific president's term of office. The terms that came out of the Watergate episode are numerous. "Détente" became a familiar word during the Nixon administration, with Kissinger's shuttle diplomacy approach to foreign affairs. President Truman's popular expression "The buck stops here" continues in use as a reference to the place where the decision-making authority resides. From the 1950s, when Senator Joseph McCarthy of Wisconsin went on an obsessive search for communist infiltration in our government, has come the term "McCarthyism." The origin and use of words provides a fascinating field for study.

Why have the innocent farm animals become symbolic of human traits? The association between the pig and police officers has already been discussed. "Turkey" was a popular label in 1976 and, again, did not convey the notion of endearment toward an individual. The word symbol turkey represents a bird that is beleaguered, unfortunate, and dumb. In fact, it is so dumb that when it looks up at the rain and opens its mouth it drowns.

However, that image, too, might convey a useful message for humans in that they, too, at times might do well to keep their mouths shut and not utter a word!

Words and sentences are not only a bundle of auditory and visual sensations but also a bundle of associations. Meaning usually is generated from *sentences* rather than from isolated words. Rearranging the words in a sentence can produce a different meaning. For example, "dog bites man" is not news, but "man bites dog" *is* news. In fact, that example serves as a guideline for reporters deciding whether or not an event is newsworthy.

Clichés are employed to convey a whole story using only a few words. "Go and boil the water" has gained universal meaning over time as symbolic of a woman who is about to have a baby and would seldom be interpreted as meaning to boil the broccoli. "The squeeky wheel gets the oil" might be paraphrased as "The complaining client gets the attention." Other trite phrases that have developed the potential to generate specific meaning are "Don't throw out the baby with the bath water," "Which comes first, the chicken or the egg?", "Six of one, half a dozen of the other," and "You get what you pay for." An immigrant who had a shoeshine stand in Central Station was asked what he had learned about America in the 40 years he had been here. His response has become a popular cliché: "There's no free lunch."

Jokes and humorous sayings mix a degree of novelty with a context that is familiar. The odd associations provide the humor; for example, "If at first you don't succeed—well so much for skydiving" or the statement, in reference to burial costs, "Returning to dust can be far from dirt cheap." Most jokes are funny because of the ridiculous nature of what is being said. The innumerable Polish jokes are classic examples.

Drawing and writing on rocks and walls, known as *graffiti*, is a form of written communication that dates back to medieval times. Today the writing is generally done in the privacy and safety of public restrooms. Graffiti is an effective means for individuals to carry on an exchange with the world and freely express what cannot be or is not expressed in everyday conversation because of personal and social constraints. It is an honest, open, gut-level expression of feelings and personal needs done without having to reveal one's identity. It provides a therapeutic effect, a catharsis of true feelings, and might even be considered one of our last media of free speech. Individuals often use graffiti to communicate their displeasure with some state of affairs and have the opportunity to vent their sexual and emotional feelings and problems. Entire books have been devoted to the description and study of graffiti.[4] The *tatoo*, or body print, differs from graffiti in that it establishes the identity of the author rather than trying to hide it.

[4]Robert George Reisner, *Graffiti: Two Thousand Years of Wall Writing*, Cowles Book Co., New York, 1971.

Controversies of all types revolve around rather obvious differences in the meaning assigned to words. In a futile effort to use words that will more likely elicit the intended meaning, we may turn to the dictionary to determine the meaning of a particular word. However, as has been said repeatedly, *there is no meaning in words themselves*; they are mere symbols used to elicit meaning. Dictionary *definitions* are of little help, for they are mere words about words, symbols about symbols. An educated adult uses about 2000 words in daily conversation. Of these, the 500 most frequently used have 14,000 dictionary definitions. Our coding system is inadequate to describe our many human experiences.

Descriptions, even humorous ones, are more adequate than definitions in eliciting the intended mental image and meaning. Some examples are as follows: "The *Golden Rule* means them that's got the gold makes the rule." "An *expert* is one who blows in, blows off, and blows out—if he is good he gets paid for it." "A *diplomat* is a person who can tell you where to go and make you look forward to the trip." "*Warm* is going barefoot in January." "A *conceited person* is the self-made man who loves his creator, or one who inflates himself with his own pump." Our language is far from exact, and word meaning resides in both the sender and the receiver of messages.

We cannot separate language from life and its occupations. Each trade and profession has its own *jargon*. Nurses seem to have a proclivity for manufacturing new words that not only divide the profession but also cause greater confusion for the consuming public. There seems to be some prestige related to coining a word and having one's name associated with it. We have copyright laws that protect one's territory of ideas, words, and trademarks. To produce new words and phrases is one thing, but more important is the ability to have them universally accepted for use with at least a close approximation of meaning between sender and receiver.

The *abbreviations* abundantly used by the health professionals are like foreign alphabet soup to the general public. The abbreviations HEW, TBC, AAA, WHO, HMO, and USPHS help speed our communication process and generally have common meaning and interpretation for individuals within the health field. However, they lack the potential to create meaning in others.

A final area to be discussed under "verbal language" and a most timely one is *sexism in language*. This subject has received increasing attention over the past 10 to 15 years, largely due to the actions of a strong feminist movement in our country. Language has played a major role in creating the stereotypes of males and females that have affected individuals' equality, potential, and freedom. Our communication patterns have fostered a male-dominated society. We have a double standard: one for males and one for females. Our should and should not systems and expectations are based on gender. For example, crying as a means of communicating emotions, while acceptable for women, is considered unacceptable for men. Biased and stereotyped expressions abound in our conversation in the home and in the business world. Women get wrinkles, but men's faces are "lined with character." A slow or erratic driver frequently is labeled a "woman driver," yet 50 percent of the time it is a man.

The development of sexist stereotypes begins in early childhood, with boys' books and toys and girls' books and toys, and is reinforced throughout our lifetime. Women's job opportunities are limited due to false assumptions and social customs that are reinforced through our language. Our mass media have been guilty of further reinforcing sexist stereotypes, but may prove to be an effective means of eradicating these inequities. A number of questions bring some of the inequities to light. Why are hurricanes only given female names? The answer is often sexist: "because they are so unpredictable." Why does a woman virtually lose her identity when she marries? She loses not only her last name but in many situations her first name as well. She becomes known and is introduced as Mrs. John Chase, not Betty Chase. Why when 89 percent of all health care providers in this country are women do these women have such a small voice in decision making relevant to health care? If a woman said "I am building a room on my cabin," it would generally be interpreted to mean that she was paying someone to make the addition. If the same statement were made by a man, he would undoubtedly be considered to be the builder. These sexist stereotypes affect our intrapersonal as well as our interpersonal communication. The intended meaning is distorted through the sexist-stereotyped glasses that are worn.

Religious organizations are experiencing great difficulty with having women accepted into roles traditionally held by men. Congregations have divided on the issue of allowing women to enter the ministry or priesthood. It is hard to believe that the role of minister, priest, or rabbi was ever male-oriented if it was based on the individual's ability. The role of the teacher, which has been predominantly held by women over the years, is not appreciably different from the comforting, supportive, counseling, and teaching role of the clergy.

Our world is cloaked in semantic expressions and semantic fallacies that have battered the self-image of women for years. The words of the past have been soaked in the past's stereotypes of women. Affirmative action programs, the Equal Rights Amendment, and all of the women's movements must and have concerned themselves with changing language to reflect the desired changes in the image of women. If we rid our communication system of these linguistic sexist patterns, individuals of both sexes should be freer and more flexible in meeting new situations.

While language has played a major role in establishing and reinforcing sexual discrimination over the years, if given proper direction it will be the powerful means by which sexual inequality can be eliminated. We must be continuously aware of the subtle as well as the gross sexual stereotypes that creep into our language. Efforts are being made to use a neuter pronoun and androgynous words that refer to both genders. Going in the other direction, such as the suggestion of replacing "history" with "herstory," will accomplish nothing. Everyone will be affected by the changes. Silverman hypothesized that as women gain more self-assertiveness, men, who previously based their masculinity on feminine servitude, will be forced to reveal themselves as inadequate individuals. He said that they will no longer be able to appear strong as they are pulled out from behind the womanly apron.[5]

It is not easy to make and accept these changes. It takes time for our nervous systems to adjust to unfamiliar symbols; for example, it is difficult to replace the "Gentlemen" or "Dear Sir" salutation with "Gentleperson" or "Dear Person." "Chairperson" is gaining popularity as a replacement for "chairman." A book that had been entitled *Hints & Tips for the Handyman* has been changed to *Hints & Tips for the Handyperson*. Although the "Manpower Administration" was not changed to the "Personpower Administration," the U.S. Department of Labor has been considering using the title "Employment and Training Administration" to more accurately portray the activities of the agency and remove reference to specific gender. Carrying through this type of thinking would require changing 3500 job titles in its *Dictionary of Occupational Titles*.

Words and the images they reflect are important to one's self-image. A high school course entitled "Home Economics for Boys" drew sparse enrollment until it was renamed. Although the course content remained the same, the new title, "Bachelor Living," drew the interest of so many students that they could not all be accommodated. Men have been asking when the labels "nurse" and "nursing" will be changed, for they produce an image not acceptable to many men at this time.

The process of ridding our communication system of linguistic or semantic bacteria is as difficult as that of gaining the universal acceptance of new words. The author painfully admits that she has not met the challenge of using neuter terms throughout this book, but promises that if subsequent editions are published, every effort will be made to meet that challenge.

NONVERBAL COMMUNICATION

Meaning can be generated from symbols other than words. Nonverbal communication involves a wide array of symbols in our body language, gestures, eye movements, facial expressions, personal appearance, and

[5]Jerome Silverman, "The Woman's Liberation Movement: Its Impact on Marriage," *Hospital and Community Psychiatry*, **26**(1):39–40, January 1975.

dress. Color and objects in our environment also have message potential. Freud pointed out how extensive our message-sending activities really are when he said: "No mortal can keep a secret. If his lips are silent, he chatters with his fingertips . . . betrayal oozes out of him at every pore."

Indian smoke signals was one of our most primitive and accurate coding systems. Our messages from the wind no longer even provide us with an accurate assessment of the direction of the wind. Man has created his own obstacles to his ability to interpret messages.

Body language is finally receiving the interest it deserves in terms of our communication behavior. The work of Birdwhistell[6] is the most prominent in the area of *kinesics*, or the study of body movement communication. Body language is our human lie detector, preventing us from concealing our inner thoughts and feelings the way we can through verbal communication. Almost 100 percent accuracy was found in diagnosing and evaluating emotionally disturbed clients through assessment of the unconscious movements of the clients' arms and legs and of the facial expressions and physical movements that accompanied the verbal responses to questions. Through the messages we send via body movement, we can convey a sense of inferiority, lack of self-confidence, or feelings of weakness or illness. Our gait and posture provide valuable clues to our self-image and self-esteem.

Veterinarians must be particularly keen in reading the body language, posture, and physical movements of sick animals. They cannot rely on verbal messages in making diagnoses, as the physician can.

We can shut off communication with others as effectively by turning our body away from them as we can by pulling the plug from a loudspeaker. These nonverbal messages are as important by themselves as they are in conjunction with verbal stimuli. We watch small children running their hands along a wall to *get in touch* with their world. Adults find it difficult to refrain from *feeling* the merchandise to add to the information about the quality and texture of the material which they received from their visual sense. We rub our eyes in the morning to get ourselves more in touch with the world. "Every little movement has a meaning all its own" are some song lyrics that reflect the importance of body language to our communication process. Man is a volume of nonverbal as well as verbal symbols if only we know how to read him. The problem is compounded when it appears that the simultaneous verbal and nonverbal messages seem to be a contradiction in meaning.

Health professionals percuss the chest and palpate the abdomen to get information about what lies hidden from view. We hit a nail with a hammer and get a message about what is below, which we hope is not a finger! The

[6]Ray L. Birdwhistell, *Kinesics and Context: Essays on Body Motion Communication,* University of Pennsylvania Press, Philadelphia, 1970.

stud finder, the x-ray, and radioactive isotopes are devices that help us gather more data upon the basis of which to make decisions. Phatic communication, or the "Hi. How are you?" is our verbal sensor, which checks the inner climate of the other individual and is used to determine whether or not interpresonal exchange is appropriate at that particular time.

Two clerks were waiting on customers at a bulk candy counter. Each clerk had a unique way of weighing the candy. The customers tended to wait in line for the one clerk rather than have the other clerk fill their order. When the first clerk was asked what she thought was the reason, she replied: "I put a small amount of candy on the scale and then *add* a little at a time until I have the amount ordered. The other clerk scoops up a lot of candy, puts it on the scale, and then *takes away* little by little until she has the desired amount." How many of us have had identical reactions, yet the message has been beyond our state of awareness?

The eyes shout what the lips fear to say. Through the expression of his eyes and eyebrows or his *eye contact* with us, we learn the degree of attention another person is showing toward us and, in some cases, his attitude toward us. The sclera helps outline the expressions of the eyes. The eyes send out accurate cues, and therefore it is not surprising that *trust* is related to an individual's ability to look one straight in the eye. Attempts have been made to attach categorical meaning to certain eye and mouth movements, yet the uniqueness of meaning cannot be overlooked. Guthrie found the mustache a means of hiding the expressions of the mouth and the man's beard a way for adult males to intimidate each other.[7] Schizophrenic and autistic children barely look at people when talking to them. The eyes serve as a valuable message source, and something seems to be missing in the exchange when one member of the party is wearing dark glasses.

"The face is the mirror of the mind, and eyes without speaking confess the secrets of the heart" (Saint Jerome). Studies have supported the theory that emotions are expressed differently across various areas of the face. The *facial expressions* of members of the audience provides important feedback to the teacher or public speaker.

Gestures are nonverbal forms used for expressing a wide variety of emotions as well as symbolic replacements for word symbols. The television comedienne Carol Burnett concludes every performance with a tug at her left earlobe as a message to her grandmother. The message meaning remains in the minds of Carol and her grandmother. However, that particular gesture is used by an Italian when sighting a pretty girl and intends to convey *appreciation*. Arabs signal appreciation of a pretty girl by stroking their beards, while Englishmen become overly casual and look

[7] R. T. Guthrie, "The Evolution of Menace," *Saturday Review*, May 1973, pp. 22–28.

away. Just as words are regionally and culturally different, so gestures also vary. When attempting to gesture that someone is *dumb*, we make a fist, extend the first finger, and move it in circles around the ear on the same side. In another country, that same intended meaning is conveyed through the gesture of taking the *right* hand, extending it over one's head, and pointing to the *left* ear.

Auctioneers rely heavily on the nonverbal gestures of potential buyers. In fact, one is afraid to even lift a finger in fear that the movement will be interpreted as a bid. Whether an individual uses a fist or an open hand in gesture has been identified as a valuable cue in the diagnosis of potential myocardial infarction victims.

Age, sex, race, and physical appearance are the first qualities noticed during a brief interpersonal encounter. Before an individual opens his mouth to speak, impressions are formed about this person from the *clothes* he wears and his general *appearance*. Clothes provide many clues to one's personality, social status, occupation, and destination. They also convey one's view of the world and one's place in it. In the past, clothes have been a good index of one's life-style and value system. As we have experienced greater freedom of dress, the information we obtain from clothing has become less reliable.

The financial state of an individual may be correctly or incorrectly inferred from his attire. For example, plaids that do not match on the side seams generally indicate less expensive clothes. We hold to many traditions in our dress. Buttons, which were originally sewed onto the sleeves of suit coats to discourage men from wiping their noses on their sleeves, remain on the sleeves today but serve more as part of the design of the garment than for any practical purpose. The original reason that men's and women's clothes buttoned in opposite directions is not known by this author, but the custom continues today. The traditional white nurse's uniform was a secular adaptation of the religious habit and was symbolic of purity. The variety of uniforms and dress worn by health care providers today serve more to identify control and one's place on the hierarchical ladder than, as is often argued, to help the consumer identify each of the numerous health care disciplines. Images and expectations are generated as associations are made between a particular uniform and a related professional discipline.

The physical appearance and dress of the client also provide valuable diagnostic cues, for they often reflect inner feelings and symptoms of illness that are not expressed verbally. Radical changes in appearance and dress are particularly useful indicators.

Our symbols appear in a myriad of *colors*, and each color leaves a different impression on our nervous system. Colors carry symbolic quality and convey some general meaning but, again, have no absolute meaning for

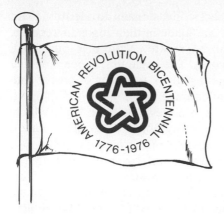

Figure 3-5   The American Bicentennial Flag.

all. Small, dark, heavy items are frequently associated with quality and value. One is left with the impression of a room being larger than it actually is when it is painted a light color. Interior decorators have been fascinated with the various color combinations and the illusions they can create. Reds generally excite, yellow is a cheerful color, greens are refreshing, purple may depress, and blues are cool colors. Color becomes our *silent salesperson* as it influences our selection.

The cover of the paperback book *Future Shock*[8] was made available in a choice of at least five colors. The choice was of no great consequence, yet the time spent in making the decision indicated that there is message meaning in those colors. The reasons behind color choice reveal something about ourselves and our internal processing of these external stimuli.

The red label of the Campbell soup can is meant to be symbolic of hot food, just as the freshness of green vegetables is to be conveyed by the Jolly Green Giant label. One disturbing feature of microwave cooking is that the food may be done but not accompanied by the rich brown color of food cooked in a conventional oven. More detailed discussion of the psychology of color is presented in an article by Haller.[9]

Organizations, states, and universities adopt *logos* as their identifying symbols. Every state has its symbolic bird, flower, and flag and every university its mascot (badger, buffalo, bear, gopher), school colors, song, and motto. The American Revolution Bicentennial Flag was a symbolic adaptation of the stars, stripes, and colors of the American flag. The symbol (Figure 3-5) is in the form of a five-pointed star in white, surrounded by continuous red, white, and blue stars that form a second star. The double star is symbolic of the two centuries that have passed since the American Revolution.

[8]Alvin Toffler, *Future Shock,* Bantam Books, New York, 1970.
[9]John M. Haller, "The Semantics of Color," *ETC*, **26**(2):201–204, June 1969.

Most organizations adopt trademarks and slogans to identify their products or services. Periodic changes are made in their logos to keep up with changes in the image they wish to create. Money is our most commonly used symbol of value and worth. The eagle that appears on the top of flagpoles and on many government seals is symbolic of power and perseverance, of virility and victory, of courage and conquest. Children, especially, have been influenced by the Smokey the Bear logo, which reminds them to be careful with matches. The symbolic tooth placed under the pillow for the fairies helps children increase their income.

The peace symbol (see Figure 3-6) was popularized during the Vietnam war by individuals who objected to United States involvement. The peace symbol's original reputation was tarnished when it became identified as the footprints of a chicken, symbolic of those who wanted peace and refused to fight.

An individual carrying a briefcase is generally thought to be a professor, salesman, or business executive and not an automobile mechanic or janitor. It has been said that years ago the Japanese businessman, in his attempt to mimic the successful American, placed only the top of the fountain pen in his top suit pocket, where it could be seen. The United States has followed the lead of the European countries by changing the word symbols on street signs to picture symbols. A great deal can be learned about an individual from studying the charms on a charm bracelet.

No institution has been so inundated with symbolism as our churches; for example, there are the symbolic water at baptism and the bread and wine as symbolic of the body and blood of Jesus. In fact, in many churches, crisp wafers have been substituted for soft bread to create a more realistic sound of breaking bread. Different colors and logos on paraments are used for each holiday and religious season. The stained glass windows depict various significant religious events.

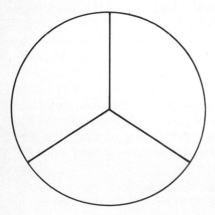

Figure 3-6 The peace symbol.

There are times when there is confusion between the spoken word and the associated visual image. Figure 3-7 is a humorous example.

Our environment is filled with objects and events that if tended to would provide us with valuable messages. The pieces of cloth hanging down from a rope stretched across two poles in a cow pasture tell me that the farmer is sensitive and considerate of his dumb animals. The apparatus is used to brush flies off of the backs of the cows as they walk under it. Ramps on curbs and at building entrances communicate concern for the handicapped. Children as well as adults have been considered when one sees high and low levels of drinking fountains. When a feeble elderly woman looks up the steep steps leading into a church, she gets the message that they do not want her there anymore. As we become sensitive to the needs of others, we communicate that concern in the buildings we construct and the environmental patterns we develop. The automobile wrecker strategically parked at a busy intersection during rush hour traffic is symbolic of the vulture awaiting its prey or of someone capitalizing on another person's misfortune.

The symbolic ground-breaking ceremony took on an interesting approach when an electronics company in Arizona was having the ceremony at the site of its new center. The dust was blowing so violently that a bucket of dirt was carried into the building next door, and the ceremony was continued as each official was allowed to turn over the dirt in the bucket.

It has been intriguing to study the location of women's restrooms in relationship to men's in public buildings. My experience has been that with few exceptions, the men's restroom comes before the women's as you go down the hall. The only explanation one might give is that this arrangement relates to the sexist and egocentric nature of the designer and the builder, who undoubtedly were men. Surely it would not be due to anything so logical as which sex has the best bladder control! One must wonder

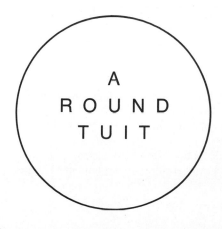

Figure 3-7 This is an indispensable item for everyone. For years people have been saying, "I'll do it as soon as I get a round tuit." On the left is a round tuit. Cut it out, keep it handy, and you will have no more trouble getting all those extras done. You finally got a round tuit.

whether these findings will change as more women enter the building trades.

The community health nurse has valuable information to assist in outlining a plan of care available to her from the client's home environment and observation of family relationships. The family also has the opportunity to obtain valuable inputs about the nurse. What does or did the nurse communicate by placing the "black bag" on newspapers, often without any explanation to the client and his family?

The musician and the artist creatively engage in symbolic thought and expression through the sounds and pictures they produce. Go to a concert and an art museum and let your mind be free to give the sounds and sights your own meaning. Too often we limit our own processing of messages as we try to have *our* meaning match that of the composer or artist. While many of the pictures bear captions, it is well not to read them until after you have assigned your own meaning.

Play therapy can be both diagnostic and therapeutic. Through drawings a client can communicate his inner feelings and frustrations. Dr. Kübler-Ross found, while studying dying children, that these children tended to use more nonverbal than verbal means of expressing their feelings. They were encouraged to draw pictures, and the pictures often depicted catastrophic events. Some children drew a stop sign, symbolic of seeking protection. The peace bird often was drawn; it was interpreted as symbolic of having come to grips with the frustrating event.[10]

Our world is truly a world of symbols. Both our verbal and our nonverbal symbols serve as messages with the potential of generating meaning and a response. We need to heighten our awareness of the nonverbal symbols especially, for they provide subtle as well as obvious messages that affect both our intrapersonal and our interpersonal communication. The effects of time and space as forms of nonverbal behavior have yet to be considered. The following chapter is devoted to the spatial-temporal dimensions, which are a significant part of all communication processes.

SUGGESTED BIBLIOGRAPHY

Boucher, Jerry D. and Paul Ekman: "Facial Areas and Emotional Information," *Journal of Communication*, **25** (2):21–29, Spring 1975.
Cundiff, Merlyn: *Kinesics: The Power of Silent Command*, Parker Publishing Co., West Nyack, N.Y., 1972.
Fast, Julius: *Body Language*, Pocket Books, Inc., New York, 1970.
Gombrich, E. H.: "The Visual Image," *Scientific American*, September 1972, pp. 82–96.

[10]Public lecture, Boulder, Colo., 1973.

Hayakawa, S. I.: *Language in Thought and Action*, 2d ed., Harcourt, Brace & World, New York, 1964.

Jakobson, Roman: "Verbal Communication," *Scientific American*, September 1972, pp. 73–80.

Langer, Susanne K.: *Philosophy in a New Key: A Study in the Symbolism of Reason, Rite and Art*, Harvard University Press, Cambridge, Mass., 1942.

Ogden, C. K. and I. A. Richards: *The Meaning of Meaning*, 8th ed., Harcourt, Brace & World, New York, 1946.

Pluckhan, Margaret L. and Charlene E. Wheeler: "Our World of Symbols," *Journal of Continuing Education in Nursing*, 3 (1):19–21, January-February 1972.

Thurman, Kelly (ed.): *Semantics*, Houghton Mifflin, Boston, 1960.

Wilson, Edward O.: "Animal Communication," *Scientific American*, September 1972, pp. 53–60.

Chapter 4

The Spatial-Temporal Dimensions of Human Communication

Love they neighbor as thyself; but don't take down the fences.

Carl Sandburg

Do not squander time for that is the stuff life *is made of.*

Benjamin Franklin

There are no nonverbal stimuli so subtle or so powerful in their potential to convey meaning as the spatial-temporal dimensions. Space and time are "silent languages" that are a part of all verbal messages. Humans exist in their environment in the here (space) and now (time). A fundamental concept of the ecologist is that *every* action, phenomenon, and move of living things is territorially based and time-oriented. Space and time provide the framework for our lives.

Time and space in and of themselves have no structure. Their significance comes from relationships. Our concern is with *duration* of time, for example, and with relative position, or *distance,* in space. From here to

there is distance, and space is the area in between. From now to then is duration, and time is the measured period in between.
We measure distance and duration, but we experience space and time as they give regularity and structure to our lives.

Each of us possesses a certain amount of space and time, and each of us varies in his need for time and space and in the ways he chooses to use them. Most if not all of the communication relative to these two dimensions concerns the issue of *control*. We seek to protect our own time and space, but we also find ourselves exerting control over the time and space of others. When we are late and others must wait, we are controlling them and the way they spend their time. When we occupy a certain space, we control it and prevent it from being occupied by others. While the spatial-temporal dimensions of communication can create a particularly difficult problem of control, the issue can be dealt with through honest communication and confrontation.

SPACE

Man is a social animal who arranges himself in physical closeness and association with others as he seeks to meet his inherent need to communicate. Space significantly affects and shapes our social interaction and interpersonal communication. The question "What are you doing here" which elicits the response "Well, everybody's got to be someplace" reflects the inherent role space plays in our lives. The sensation of space involves a synthesis of visual, auditory, kinesthetic, olfactory, and thermal sensory inputs.

We are constantly arranging ourselves in this universe in some spatial order in relation to other people and objects. Sometimes we have the freedom to occupy the space we want, to have a degree of solitude and psychological distance from others if we wish it. At other times we are forced to exist in a physical area so confining and crowded that we experience physical and psychological disturbances. We may experience *claustrophobia*, or the morbid dread of closed or narrow places. The fear of heights, often experienced by the tourist on his first trip to the mountains, is a fear of the extreme opposite spatial relationship. The person who is frightened of heights elects to sit in the middle of the car seat, with other people seated on both sides, in an effort to psychologically break the spatial distance into fragments his nervous system can tolerate.

"Why do you climb mountains?" is a question frequently asked of mountain climbers. A common response is that it gives one an exalted feeling as one looks down and around into the open space. Another response expresses ambivalence between feeling "free as a bird" and not being confined by people or buildings and perceiving self as truly insignificant in relation to the massive and uninterrupted environment below. For some mountain climbers, the reason may be the sheer joy of conquering distance. Whatever the answer, the spatial dimension is inherent in it.

Extensive studies relating to space and territoriality are long past due. In recent years, primarily due to our population explosion and its threatening consequences, we have been forced to become more concerned about limitations of space. People are not the only inhabitants of space. A frightening statistic from as far back as 1966 revealed that 60 to 70 percent of the space in Los Angeles was devoted to automobiles. Crowding, whether from objects or from people, disrupts social relationships and affects communication. Illness and crime have been traced to crowded conditions. "Green belts" have been set aside in large metropolitan areas to attempt to offset the plethora of man-made structures and buildings that damage our nervous system. As increased crowding becomes evident, architects are working to at least give the illusion of more freedom in our use of space. The buildings designed by the well-known architect Frank Lloyd Wright attest to that fact.

Space is essentially that *nothingness* that exists between self at the point of departure and some object or person perceived in the "world out there." In this respect, space is undoubtedly the most significant "nothing" we have. It has been referred to as "room to move about in" or "a place to put our bodies in." To be aware of space is to be aware of the invisible. Much as Elwood was aware of and affected by his invisible rabbit, Harvey, and as a doctor must be aware of and appreciate the importance of an invisible virus, so the communicator must be aware of the effect the dimension of space has on both his intrapersonal and his interpersonal communication processes. We must yield to the powers and demands imposed upon us by the nonhuman nonentity labeled "space."

Space is involved in our communication process in three ways: (1) as an internal message source, (2) as an external, nonverbal message, and (3) as noise on the communication channel which affects the message.

As an *internal* message source, space serves as a symbolic construct with the power to generate meaning and communication with the person himself. Through the self-reflexive quality of humans, a thought may trigger a sensation of space and evolve into a fear of heights or anger about crowding. An individual may sense a spontaneous response to his self-generated and space-related stimulus without either an external message source or other individuals being involved. As man creates his own reality, space becomes one dimension of that world.

Space as an *external*, nonverbal message source can affect both our intrapersonal and our interpersonal communication. Most individuals can tolerate a small office if they can push their chair back from the desk without hitting anything. The distance a person senses between an object in the office and himself is an example of intrapersonal communication with a space-related external stimulus. When that same individual leaves the office and positions his body in relation to another individual, he becomes involved in interpersonal communication in which external, nonverbal spatial messages are potentially sensed stimuli. Distance is present in *all* interpersonal encounters in varying degree. Our language of space is in juxtaposition to our verbal language. For example, the loudness of our verbalization is adjusted in relation to our perception of the distance between and among members in the interaction. We may say things at a distance which we would not say in a face-to-face confrontation. Most of us must admit that on occasion we have uttered words only after a person has turned to walk away. The written memo may be consciously or unconsciously used to keep distance between sender and receiver, to prevent an immediate feedback or response. Sending messages through a third party is another way to either extend or attempt to reduce the distance between individuals as they communicate. For example, "Johnny, tell your mother I don't have time to change the furnace filter now" may be using Johnny as a mediator or as an impersonal object to maintain distance from the other person. The context or situation in which the statement was made will be influencial in assessing the intended message meaning.

Edward T. Hall, an anthropologist, was a pioneer in the conceptualization and study of space in interpersonal relationships.[1] He used the term *proxemics* to describe the theories of man's use of space. For people in our Western culture, Hall described the following four interpersonal distance zones: (1) *Intimate distance* includes the important area of touch but generally involves a 6- to 18-inch space between people. (2) *Personal distance* is within arm's reach of one another and generally is 1½ to 4 feet. (3) *Social distance* is 4 to 12 feet and is most often used in business activities. (4) *Public distance* is 12 to 25 or more feet and is generally found between a public speaker or entertainer and his audience.[2] Within these zone norms, variations exist depending upon the specific activity, setting, and general relationship between individuals in the interaction. The language of space is difficult to interpret, for as Hall stated, "The fact that the message conveyed is couched in no formal vocabulary makes things doubly difficult, because neither party can get very explicit about what is actually taking place."[3]

Each culture has acceptable standards for its language of space. We master a culture, and before we realize it that culture has controlled us with its norms, codes, system of values, and rituals. The patterns and bound-

---

[1]Edward T. Hall, *The Silent Language,* Fawcett Publishers, Greenwich, Conn., 1959.
[2]Edward T. Hall, *The Hidden Dimension,* Doubleday & Co., Garden City, N.Y., 1966, pp. 109–120.
[3]Hall, *The Silent Language,* p. 19.

aries of space are learned informally and most often are totally out of our awareness. The great mobility of people between continents has given us a mix of cultures, a confusing array of proxemics, and inevitable cross-cultural communication problems. Misevaluations are to be expected as messages are encoded in one cultural context and decoded in another. Although cultural patterns are in a constant state of flux, it takes generations for cultural differences to actually disappear.

The concept of *touch*, the most intimate distance, is a topic worthy of an entire volume. It is interesting to note that small children freely touch one another and sit or stand in closer proximity to each other than adults do. A young child learns to associate security with the closeness conveyed by touch. As he matures, he finds that he must alienate himself from this close contact with his mother and others as he strives for independence. People in our culture generally are adverse to touching. In fact, if someone touches or bumps us accidently, a quick apology is made. How many people have you communicated with today through the language of touch? Was the touch intentional? What response did it elicit from the receiver? Have you ever witnessed the "dance" between two people with different limits to their spatial distance? One moves in as he speaks, the other backs off, and the first person advances again to reduce the spatial distance between them. It is a dialogue without words and might be called the "proxemic dance."

Touch is one of our most vivid means of expression. It has the power to enhance the transmission of meaning from a verbal message. Tactile channels may be open when the verbal one is blocked, as when we are trying to get someone's attention. Because touch is a more spontaneous form of communication, it generally is more authentic than verbal communication and is the most accurate form.

The distance from another person that we sense may be in no way related to measured physical distance. Shake hands with three individuals: What kind of message meaning did you perceive from each one? Many handshakes convey a sense of great distance rather than the sense of intimacy that the touch might be expected to convey. Conversely, we can experience intimacy even from a distance. A word, a smile, a wink, or steady eye contact may bring even a public distance of 12 feet within the sensed distance of 6 to 18 inches.

The individuals involved and the context or situation dictate acceptable distance zones. How often when walking toward a stranger or even an associate on the sidewalk do we glance down and lose eye contact as we get into the personal or intimate distance zones! Each of us has his own tolerance for closeness and distance in addition to our cultural patterning. It is acceptable in our culture for a male and female to touch and hold hands, but it is less acceptable for two of the same sex to do it. Some of these cultural patterns relating to interpersonal spacing are undergoing changes. The barefoot era was intended in part as a means by which individuals could *get in touch with the world*, feel and be sensitive to the various stimuli in our environment. The irony of it was that frequently the barefoot individuals got into their automobiles, with their huge, wide, soft tires, to eliminate the "feel" or bumps in the road.

Noise on a communication channel is anything on the channel other than what the communicator put there. Because space is such an invisible and subtle construct, it often is unintentional and out of awareness of the sender but appears as noise and an obstructing force that causes much confusion and uncertainty.

Although not part of the intended message, spatial noise can serve as a competing message that affects the communication in varying degrees. It may be so powerful as to replace an intended verbal message or so subtle and weak as to cause only minor concern on the part of the receiver. An example of a strong space-related disturbance would be having the verbal statement "I'm not afraid of contracting your disease" be accompanied by the speaker standing a substantial distance from the receiver. Confusion and uncertainty result when verbal and nonverbal spatial messages are not perceived as congruent. Which message is most influential will depend upon the strength of the signal as well as the psychological set of the individual at that particular time and in that particular setting. We read meaning into the way people behave as much as into what they verbalize. Actions generally *do* speak louder than words.

Territoriality is the drive to gain, maintain, and defend one's exclusive right to an area of space or piece of property. Territorial behavior has been identified and studied in bird and animal life for some time. Robert Ardrey, an anthropologist and playwright, recently has expressed his belief that humans also exhibit territorial behavior in both inward compulsions and overt acts as they seek to possess and defend space. He has further proposed that the territorial nature of man is both genetic and ineradicable. As humans, according to Ardrey, we compete and fight for both physical and psychological space. Territoriality is a human biological need, it is imperative, and we cannot control it, for it is instinctively based. It motivates all human beings.[4]

Many explanations have been proposed for this territorial drive of humans. Some theorists claim that food is the basis upon which man seeks and defends space. Others hypothesize that territoriality is sexually based. Ardrey used his playwright's wit when he said that the notion of romance was killed when Howard discovered, when studying bird life, that male birds seldom quarrel over females, but usually over real estate. It was

[4]Robert Ardrey, *The Territorial Imperative,* Atheneum Publishers, New York, 1966.

Ardrey's belief that the reason humans strive to acquire and defend territory is that territory provides the means whereby all three basic human needs can be met simultaneously. He characterized these needs as *identity, stimulation,* and *security.* The more territory is compressed, the greater the fight to preserve it.[5]

Each species of lower animal has its own means of identifying its territorial boundaries, checking on intruders, and displaying aggressive behavior toward trespassers. Dogs urinate in strategic areas to mark their claim and sniff to determine if others have invaded their turf. Deer leave a scent from glandular secretions, and monkeys vocalize their territorial rights. The beaver uses musk oil to stake its claim.

The territorial behavior displayed by humans is more civilized but also more elaborate and extensive. Our environment is inundated with symbols devised by humans to identify territorial bounds. We have "no trespassing" signs, name plates on desks, labels on clothes, copyrights, and legal deeds to property. We have zoning laws and restrictive covenants to help preserve the quality of the territory as well as the property itself. We grow hedges and build walls. In the city of Denver, fences are the rule rather than the exception. One must ponder whether the purpose of fences is to keep someone or something *in* or someone or something *out.* Some residents further protect their property with a "Beware of Dog" sign.

We also lay claim to objects; for example, we identify the ownership of a chair by placing a coat or other object on it. We even lay claim to layers of property, one person owning the property, another the mineral rights. As solar energy is starting to be used to heat homes, legislation is being written to protect one's space of sunlight from being obstructed by trees and buildings. Humans as well as animals respond to intrusions of their territory with aggressive behaviors, including verbal accusations, overt acts, and physical attacks.

Even though Ardrey believed in the instinctual nature of territorial behavior in humans, he also recognized the influence of culture and other factors. Just as we are prisoners of the spoken word, so also are we prisoners of our cultural conditioning, which is superimposed upon our innate need to seek and defend territory. In American culture, we think nothing of moving chairs and furniture around to claim physical space. But the German culture looks upon such behavior as a violation of mores. The Japanese use a single room for many activities, whereas the Americans have separate rooms for dining, sleeping, and playing. In rooms where there are no discrete and obvious room divisions, we may find plant, wood, or curtain dividers. Some cultures place the furniture in the center of the

[5] Ardrey, *The Territorial Imperative.*

room, while others, like ours, place it on the periphery of each room. We handle space as we converse with others, as we carry on our business activities, and as we plan buildings and arrange furniture. Winston Churchill put it most appropriately when he said, "We shape our buildings and then they shape us."

The territorial concept is evident in our personal and social lives. When seated in a theater, haven't you wondered if the chair arm to your right or left "belonged" to you? Haven't you ever drawn an imaginary line down a shared desk or dresser? Haven't you become upset when two or three individuals walked abreast on the sidewalk and forced you off "your" half of the walk? How do you feel when someone's cigarette smoke flows into "your" airway? Obviously the territorial drive is a motivating force behind efforts to restrict smoking in increasing numbers of our public buildings. What is your reaction to someone whose anatomy hangs over into "your" seat on an airplane? How do you feel when you spot a parking space, quickly label it "yours," and then have someone slip into the space ahead of you? What is your territorial response to someone who takes the classroom seat you have had for the full semester? We so habitually return to the same seat that it was not very surprising when one of the students came up to me after class and asked if he could be assigned to a different seat. The irony of the question was that no formal seating assignments had ever been made in that class. He obviously had confused external constraints with constraints of his own making. It was true although hard to believe that in a small mountain town where snow seems to fall by the foot at times, an individual became so upset at having to shovel the snow that had drifted from his neighbor's property that he colored "his" snow to claim *his* property.

As we stand in the coffee line at work, in a tow line on the ski slope, or in the supermarket checkout line, we recognize the many territorial claims that are so much a part of a civilized society. Our physical and psychological worlds are full of real and imaginary territorial boundary lines. Limited physical space can interfere with one's ability to get the required psychological space. The mother and five children who have outgrown the house experience daily interpersonal communication problems.

It requires a secure person and open communication to view privacy as a need rather than reading it as a rejection or a withdrawal. In some families, husband and wife symbolize their need for privacy by wearing specific head pieces. One husband wore a golf hat when he wanted his own space for a while, and the wife wore a bandana to signify a need to have here own territory. In some university dormitories where it was a habit for students to trespass in one another's private rooms, the policy adopted was that a bath towel be hung on the outside doorknob of the room when intrusion by others was less than welcome. Everyone has a need for his personal and private space for thinking, feeling, and communicating with self.

Family therapy is based in part on the notion that problems of interaction patterns are related to quarrels over territory. At retirement, problems often develop between husband and wife as the husband is home more and invades the wife's previously claimed territory during certain hours of the day. "I like my husband home—but not for lunch" clearly points to territorial needs that will lead to discord if not met.

Our environment places many spatial constraints on our growth. If a flower is planted in a pot, it will grow to the limits of that pot. Plant the same flower in a field and it will take on a totally different character. So it is with individuals. We need freedom and space to expand and grow to the limits of our capabilities.

We not only have a unique system for defending property but also have innovative ways of rearranging space to best meet our needs. Our increasing paucity of space requires a reallocation of it and a discovery of more profitable means for using this necessary element. Skyscrapers and high-rise apartment buildings are being constructed in increasing numbers to make use of vertical space when horizontal space is at a premium. Even our topography is being changed, as hills are being leveled, mountains lowered, marshes drained, and oceans filled. Flying has become a welcome alternative to traveling on crowded highways. Other ways in which we attempt to rearrange ourselves in space are suggested in an article entitled "Space: The Silent Language. . . ."[6]

As we become crowded in our limited space, our desire for private ownership of land increases. We come to view property as one way to keep some sense of freedom, independence, and control. Humans tend to become more irritable, more competitive, and less tolerant of others when they experience crowded conditions. Physical and emotional illness, violence, and crime result.

At the other end of the continuum from crowding is confinement or isolation. All of these have effects on behavior. While we have limits on our tolerance for excessive inputs resulting from overcrowding, we must have inputs for stimulation. Each of us must study our own response to such spatial conditions as lack of privacy, confinement, and crowding. We can learn about ourselves and how the spatial dimension affects us by going out in a crowd, climbing a mountain, or sitting in the quiet countryside.

Humans extend their territorial behavior to social as well as physical territory. Social territoriality is particularly important to life in the United States. The study of communication in groups has led to interest in the

[6]Margaret L. Pluckhan, "Space: The Silent Language . . ." *Nursing Forum,* **VII**(4): 386–397, 1968.

concept of social territory. Humans are possessive of objects, ideas, and cognitive turf; of other people; of status; even of words. We defend our social status and challenge others as we attempt to better ourselves. The rungs of the territorial ladder might be said to be traveled by "social climbers." The drive to achieve status is an internal pressure to achieve dominance over social partners. Interpersonal communication plays a principal role in our efforts to seek status among our peers. The distance maintained in a social interaction is often symbolic of the power structure, or power among the group members. Studies have shown a correlation between interpersonal distance and social rank. The physical space assigned to employees in an organization is dependent upon the position and status of the occupants and not on the actual space needed to get work done. The fact that the office space assigned is related to the hierarchical pecking order is no accident.

Our verbal language is loaded with possessive pronouns. We use "my" to claim ownership of people as well as of objects. Establishing territorial claim to other people as well as to physical property can be a dangerous game for both the possessor and the possessed. We frequently find that husbands who have been divorced from "their" wives become enraged and exhibit aggressive behavior when they see their former wives in the company of other men.

A final important aspect of territoriality is how we lay claim to and defend a work area. We have an unlimited number of trade unions that were set up in part to help protect specific jobs and areas of employment. As consumers if not as providers of health care, we should be concerned about the quality of that care. Many of our major problems in our health care delivery system are either directly or indirectly related to "professional territoriality."[7] Efforts to effectively coordinate the galaxy of health care professionals needed to provide care are often hampered by actions of professionals fearful that other professional groups will trespass upon their claimed territory of practice. Although the license to practice nursing or medicine has as its primary purpose protecting the public from incompetents, the license is used to protect and preserve certain roles and responsibilities for a select segment of health professionals. *Right of passage* is a phrase used by anthropologists to mean off limits to others than those specified. The drive by one professional group to prevent the encroachment of professionals from other health care disciplines into their claimed territorial boundaries has served to stifle efforts to deliver effective and coordinated health care to consumers.

Professionals are not alone in their struggle for territory within the health care system. Utterances in defense of the status quo by hospital

[7]Margaret L. Pluckhan, "Professional Territoriality: A Problem Affecting the Delivery of Health Care," *Nursing Forum,* **XI**(3): 300–310, 1972.

administrators are being heard across the country. The administrators have found that the surgicenter concept, Health Maintenance Organizations (HMOs), ambulatory care centers, and neighborhood health stations threaten their past claims to client-population territory and the income related to it. Change is a real threat to ownership, and the aggressive behavior observed is evidence of the important role social, as well as physical, territoriality plays. Physicians who over the years have fought everything from the use of the bathtub to group practice to the general practitioner to Medicare and now National Health Insurance and the nurse practitioner programs have been reflecting territorial behavior. Nurses are fighting to keep physician assistants and other ancillary personnel from infringing on their territorial domain. One must wonder whether the nurse/doctor fight over professional territory is not also a female/male control issue.

Psychologists and sociologists have been highly critical of the theories proposed by Ardrey[8] regarding territoriality in humans. They claim that his theories are unfounded; yet Ardrey has conducted more research in the area to support his thesis than they have to support theirs. The irony of the dispute is that Ardrey, an anthropologist, may be viewed as intruding into *their* professional territory. The reader is encouraged to study an interesting dialogue between Ardrey in his book *The Social Contract*[9] and writings in the book entitled *Man and Aggression*.[10]

TIME

The temporal dimension has much in common with the spatial one when we attempt to describe it and explore the part it plays in the communication process. Both are nonentities yet are highly operative and significant. Time and space are both conditions of our thinking and communicating with ourselves and others. Time may not be a tangible object, but the sensed reality of our experiences with it cannot be denied. Time is a concept, an experience, and a way of perceiving. How we spend time becomes an important question in our lives. A glaring social problem that confronts us is how to spend our increased leisure time.

Verbal messages with reference to time are etched in the verb tense used. The tense indicates whether the content refers to past, present, or future. Our political affiliations have a temporal dimension. The label "liberal" carries the connotation of speedy advance and change while "conservative" implies delay and maintaining the status quo. Our verbal

    [8]Ardrey, *The Territorial Imperative*.
    [9]Robert Ardrey, *The Social Contract,* Atheneum Publishers, New York, 1970
    [10]M. F. Ashley Montagu (ed.), *Man and Aggression,* Oxford University Press, New York, 1968.

language contains a wealth of time-oriented words, such as "now," "later," "soon," "year," "month," "hour," and "season." We also have time-related phrases, such as "from time to time," "at times," and "in no time." New Year's Day and July 4 are examples of specific time. Shakespeare was particularly fond of the word "time," and it appears in many of his works.

Time also enters our communication as an intended message on the nonverbal level. It may appear alone as a nonverbal message or accompany verbal language and serve as redundancy in an effort to help get the message across to the receiver. For example, an individual may say that he does not want to go to a party and then reinforce that verbal message by arriving late. We may eat dinner late in the evening to communicate, by symbolic use of time, that we are "fashionable."

The temporal dimension may also function as *noise* on the communication channel. We are all familiar with the long-winded speaker whose message becomes clouded and eventually fades from our perception as time moves on. The breakdown in communication between the speaker and his audience may be misinterpreted as being caused by verbal language rather than nonverbal noise. Most of the time, a long-winded speaker is unaware that he is sending a loud unintentional message that is becoming noise to the audience.

We cannot dissociate ourselves from time. It is the essential ingredient that gives order to our lives and allows us to coexist with one another in our society. Life is filled with rhythms and cycles of time.

Our experience with time has both beneficial and detrimental effects. Time is the coordinating unit that allows people to work, play, and live together. In our society we need to have some simultaneity in our actions, some standardized times for attending classes, for playing bridge, for attending church, and for starting and finishing work. Traffic lights are timed to regulate the flow of traffic and reduce the chaos and the accidents that would result from uncontrolled movement of traffic. However, time patterns are frequently so restrictive that they prevent flexibility in our lives and stifle creativity. Humans place many temporal pressures upon themselves. The result is stomach ulcers, heart disease, hypertension, and a variety of other psychosomatic ills. It is the perfectionist who has a high regard for time who "takes great pains and also gives and gets them."

Time is of prime importance in our industrial world. Machines are timed to coordinate, pace, and even control man and his work. We have budgets of time as well as of money. The Program Evaluation and Review Technique, commonly known as PERT, relies heavily on the temporal dimension in its programmed plan for coordinating unrelated activities to meet preassigned deadlines and phases of work. Business organizations as well as individuals set time-oriented goals. Organizations capitalize on the ability of computers to provide instant financial information, which allows for the immediate investment of assets; to these organizations time saved is money earned.

Our perception of time is affected by the occupation we choose. Some positions automatically call for greater concern for time and adherence to time schedules than others do. In health care facilities in particular, time schedules exert powerful control over our activities. We have a galaxy of symbols, such as qid, tid, and q 2 hr, to facilitate the process.

We sense both the *passing of time (motion)* and the *length of time (duration)*. Time moves through the *past-present-future triad*. Our unique time-binding capacity allows us to use the retained past as well as present information in the future. Even during vacations, we are aware of the passing of time, of what day it is, what time of day it is, and what part of the vacation remains before we must return to work.

We live along a time continuum from birth to death. The effects the passing of time have on us are indicated by the lucrativeness of the cosmetic industry, with its hair dyes, rejuvenation powders, and wrinkle creams to help us deceive ourselves and others into thinking that time stands still and we are not growing old. In conversation, we tend to refer to the longest portion of our lives. Below the age of 40 we generally talk about the future, while after that time, we generally refer to the past. There is a marked change in how we experience time as we grow older. Many of our communication problems occur across generational lines for that reason. When a young person wants change, he generally means *now*, not within the next 5 years. We also tend to sense time as passing quickly or slowly depending upon the urgency and significance we place upon the event.

Time is dynamic: people, objects, and events change over time. The message in a restaurant window attests to that fact: "No need to say grace over our hash—it was blessed as roast beef yesterday."

As has been discussed previously, *memory*, which entails the preservation of the past, is a crucial part of the entire intrapersonal communication process. Events are located in memory, and we recall them sequenced in time frames. We cannot escape the past, for it continously shapes our present and future ideas and activities. Dreams are viewed by some observers as being experiences with the yet unlived future. Others theorize that dreams are the result of confusion of the three time frames on the continuum. We all know the discontent of individuals who live most of their lives in the past and do little to advance themselves or the society in which they live.

It is inconceivable for those of us who have great concern for the future to believe that many people do not hold it in such awe. To the Navajo Indians, for example, only the immediate has reality. The mystical and unpredictable nature of the future is pushed aside, and plans for the future are not worth thinking or talking about. The Pueblo Indians have no set time for events. They start an activity when the time is ripe and not before. The Arabs look back 2000 to 6000 years when discussing the past.

We perceive *duration* in relationship to varied activities and our ability to see change. When totally involved in something that interests us or gives us pleasure, we often lose track of time. How urgent the event is, whether one is engaged in more than one thing at a time, whethere or not one is busy, and how much variety enters into the situation all affect one's sensation of duration of time. The sense of duration may be lost when there are no windows through which to see events changing in the world outside. Duration takes its toll of healthy relationships, for "company, like fish, spoil after 5 days."

We attribute meaning to 20 minutes or 1 hour of lateness and respond accordingly. A mother may overlook a 5-minute wait for her child, but she may become irritated with the child after waiting 20 minutes and would undoubtedly be worried as well as irritated after waiting 1 hour.

Much of our communication relating to time is culturally based and controlled. For example, people from Latin American countries accept much longer waits than do Americans, who are generally incensed with delays. Punctuality is a highly regarded American middle-class value. Lateness often implies indifference, an insult, and/or irresponsibility. It may also be interpreted as lack of interest, as lack of appreciation for and sensitivity to time or to you as a person.

Cross-cultural differences concerning time provide us with many problems. For example, a Spanish American may be functioning according to the belief system *"Mañana es bastante bueno para me"* ("Tomorrow is good enough for me") while the Caucasion working with him is operating under the notion "Don't put off for tomorrow what you can do today." When we use time words, of which there are many in our culture, we must be aware of and sensitive to how each is perceived. Some cultures actually view punctuality as rudeness and bad manners. Rules of etiquette dictate that one arrive 5 minutes late so as not to convey eagerness. Lateness is an offense on some occasions and in some cultures.

We have innumerable examples in our culture of roles that carry a time dimension along with their activity. The white-collar worker generally begins his working day later than the general laborer. For years there was and there may still exist an implied rule that a student was obligated to wait 15 minutes for a full professor, 10 minutes for an associate professor, and 5 minutes for an assistant professor. The instructor and the student were expected to be on time.

For some individuals a norm is broken when they are called at home on a Sunday about business matters. A phone call at 3 A.M. is often experienced with anxiety, for it is interpreted as an urgent situation. Lack of clear norms on temporal matters causes misevaluation and results in tension in interpersonal relationships. "A little while" for one person may be a "long time" for another. Time is not absolute, but relative. Punctuality may be viewed with indifference and as an irrational expectation by some people but be sensed as a totally rational expectation by others, who consider a 5-minute lateness by one individual who keeps six people waiting as robbing those individuals of a total of 30 minutes of valuable time. From early childhood each of us has to some degree been conditioned relative to the meaning of time to us.

We have four timing mechanisms available to us for checking time reality. We have inner physiological and psychological timing and outer ecological and technological measures of time.

Our biological clock—our inherent timing mechanism—is responsible for various cyclic physiological and behavioral responses. Our *physiological timers* involve our nervous system, which registers time durations and communicates messages regarding such bodily needs as hunger, thirst, and the like. Our *psychological timing* involves our feelings and sensations of the passing and duration of time. These are influenced by the particular activities and individuals involved in the process. "When I am with you time goes so fast" is a statement of psychological time sensation. Time appears to move faster when we are enjoying ourselves. When someone is sad or depressed, he may withdraw and go to sleep in an effort to speed the passing of inner time.

We organize time into divisions of work, play, and sleep. Our physiological and psychological timing mechanisms attempt to force us to maintain a healthy balance. We wed time and specific activities throughout the day and throughout our lives. We divide our day into mealtime points of reference, referring to activities to be done "before breakfast," "after lunch," or "before dinner." Obvious confusion and misinterpretation arise when dinner refers to a noon meal to some people and to an evening meal to others.

Man is a living clock and can maintain himself through his inner timing devices. However, to obtain the uniformity in our timing which is essential to coordinating activities with others, *external timing devices* are required. Our *ecological timers* are the sun and the moon. The body's shadow made by the sun was the human sundial. The hand dial, a portable sundial, was devised in order for people to be more exact as to the hour of the day. In ancient days the sundial fired a gun to announce midday. In some of our cities, this tradition persists but the shot has been replaced with a loud horn or whistle. The astrolabe came into use both for observing the stars and as a timekeeping device. Time telling was limited to daylight hours with previous measuring devices, but night hours could be determined with the astrolabe, which used the "pointer" stars of the Great Bear constellation.

Most sundials contain some philosophical statement about the passing of time. The following one that is common and was written by Longfellow: "What is time?—The shadow on the dial, the striking of the clock, the running of the sand, day and night, summer and winter, months, years, centuries—these are but the arbitrary and outward signs, the measure of Time, not Time itself. Time is the life of the soul."

Although time is invisible, the visual and *mechanical timing devices* called "clocks" and "calendars" which man has constructed serve to make us more aware of its duration and passing. An unpretentious investigation of three households consisting of two adults each was made to determine how many man-made timing devices they contained. The average per household was 16, which included clocks, watches, calendars, and other timing devices. If this sample is typical of most households, and if the number of devices signifies the importance of time in our lives, the findings speak for themselves. Priestley said, "Clock time is our bank manager, tax collector, police inspector; inner time is our wife."[11]

Man's genius and concern for time are exemplified by a study of attempts to develop mechanized and standardized means to uniformly measure and record time. The calendar and clock are our most useful external timing devices. The calendar is much the same today as when it was first introduced in 46 B.C. It became known as the "Gregorian calendar" after slight changes were made by Pope Gregory XIII in 1593. In religious circles it helped to regulate feasts and temple services. It has been theorized that many Jewish boys grew up to be great mathematicians because of the amount of computation needed to interpret the Jewish calendar.

A brief overview of the history and development of clocks reflects the motivation and creative ability of man as it relates to time. In 1276, the mercury clock, using cogs linked to a rod, came into prominence. The fourteenth century brought with it mechanical clocks based on the principle of falling weights tied to a rope around a revolving drum. This is the principle behind our present-day cuckoo and grandfather clocks. In the fifteenth century, the hourglass, or ships' "watch," was developed. It contained powdered marble boiled in wine. Even at that time, marked candles and oil were burned to symbolize and correspond to the passing of time. In 1581 Galileo discovered the principle of the pendulum, which would later be used in mechanized clocks.

In the seventeenth century, the sandglass was first used to time sermons. The story was told of how children would watch the time pass as the sand flowed from one glass to the other and were disappointed when the preacher would turn the sandglass over to flow for an additional 60 minutes.

[11]J. B. Priestley, *Man and Time,* Doubleday & Co., Garden City, N.Y., 1964, p. 66.

This is not unlike the practice of students today, who estimate the amount of time remaining by the amount of film remaining on the reel when a film is being shown. The egg timer used in many homes today is a replica of the early sandglass timing device. A story was told about a widow who, when asked what she intended to do with her husband's ashes, replied that she would put them into an egg timer. "Lazy beggar," she said, "would never work when he was alive, he can do summet now he's dead."

In the same seventeenth century, hair or balance springs were used to lighten the mechanism in the clock and thereby made the portable pocket watch possible. In 1840 the electric clock was invented, and it opened a wide avenue of timing possibilities. The number and diversity of timing apparatuses on our electrical appliances are well known to all. In addition to the visual sensation of the passing of time, the "tick-tock" sound of the clock audibly reinforces in our minds the fluid state of time.

Our elaborate system of timing devices has brought a degree of order into our lives and helped avoid the inevitable chaos that would occur without these devices. We have become a clock-ridden society and are suffering from "temporal constipation." While the need for uniform referent time frames cannot be disputed, we have virtually succumbed to the dictates of the clock. Although man-made timing devices were intended to supplement our physiological timing mechanisms, clock time dominates our inner time and controls our functioning. Yet it takes only an electrical power failure, that upsets our time schedule for that day when the electric alarm clock does not go off as intended, especially one, during our sleeping hours, to renew our appreciation for timing devices and the role they play in our lives.

Clock time tells us when we should eat, and calendar time dictates the age at which we must retire. Only the infant has the privilege of eating when his *physiological* inner clock says he wants or needs food. From then on we succumb to the *mechanical* outer clock, which dictates our eating habits and literally tells us when we should be hungry. We have bells ring and whistles blow, as Pavlov did with his dog, to tell us when to start salivating.

We cannot change outer time but only the inner sensation of time. If one is bored and/or engaged in an unpleasant task, time may appear to be moving slowly. Watching the hands on the clock move is analogous to watching the pot, which never boils. Our inner timing mechanism is not necessarily attuned to clock time. The greatest difficulty experienced by individuals who have tried to live buried underground was their miscalculation of time. Mental illness often includes a temporal disorientation. Memory is lost when an individual is unable to build a relationship in time. When we change to daylight saving time, our inner sensations and external activities must be readjusted.

Although we share outer or clock and calendar time, inner time is an individual matter. Some people have a particularly accurate sense of inner time as it relates to outer time. These individuals feel comfortable without having to rely upon a wristwatch or an alarm clock. We have our own notion of how much can be accomplished by us in a certain time frame. More often than not this estimate is unrealistic. Individualized perception as it relates to time takes a toll on interpersonal communication.

Everyone is entitled to at least one pet peeve, and being an acknowledged time-oriented person, one of mine is the albatross in our health care system known as the "waiting room." The abominable "wait" sends a nonverbal message that is not in the best interest of either the consumer or the provider of health care. Having someone wait is viewed not only as inconsiderate and disrespectful but as controlling as well. Certainly in the health field one should reasonably expect that respect will be shown for the person and his possessions. One of man's most valuable possessions is *time*.

Probably no physical space in the environment in which health care is given is more appropriately labeled than the waiting room—for waiting it is! At least the consumer is not deceived by a label "guest room," "reception room," or "admitting room" instead of "waiting room." A waiting room might well be defined as a space where large numbers of clients congregate. They often must sit on uncomfortable furniture inappropriately arranged and have access to old and well-used magazines. Each client is there to meet with the doctor or receive health care at a definite and prearranged time (an explicit contract between the client and agency or health worker). The irony of the contract is that it seems to be binding to only one of the parties—the client. The health care personnel do not seem to be obligated to respect the time schedule of the contract, but the client is expected to conform. Therefore it is not surprising to have the client feel insignificant as a person and sense *his* time as an unimportant concern of others.

A study of the origin and history of the waiting room in health care facilities would be an interesting one. One might expect that waiting rooms started a long time ago, when the horse-and-buggy doctor spent hours traveling to visit patients and deliver babies and the clinic staff had few guidelines to follow in estimating how long it would take him to return for his scheduled appointments. Today, with rapid and much more predictable forms of transportation available to clients and doctors alike, one can estimate with relative accuracy how long it will take to get to the office. The physician *should* be able, after years of "practice," to arrive at a predictable average time needed for each clinic visit. Why then do waiting rooms and the indignities associated with them persist?

The wait has become endemic in our society and is a social disease, an interpersonal communication problem, which we can and must irradicate. It produces symptoms of anger, distrust, anxiety, and frustration. Is it any wonder that clients, who must routinely wait for scheduled appointments, feel a sense of worthlessness as they spend valuable time and money to obtain health care? Ask any health care consumer what his greatest complaint is and the "frustrations of having to wait for appointments" ring through loud and clear.

Emergencies are expected on the health care scene and will cause delays in meeting schedule appointments, but these are not the reason for most delays. A study by Johnson and Rosenfeld[12] of the length of waiting among eight ambulatory care facilities showed wide variations. They found that slightly under one-half of the 3590 clients in the study waited an hour or more. Eight percent had to wait only 10 minutes or less, and 13 percent waited 2 or more hours. These findings were contrasted with an English study that showed that only 11 percent of the 12,477 clients observed had to wait an hour or more to see the doctor. Both studies identified the same two basic causes for clients having to wait, namely, lateness of the doctor and poor design of the appointment system.

The practice of having clients wait has become a habit and a routine in hospitals and emergency rooms as well as in private clinics. In fact, one of the original reasons for developing the intensive care unit as part of the total progressive patient care concept was to bypass the admitting procedure and admit the clients directly to the unit. If the expected wait could be avoided, care could be initiated more rapidly and lives could be saved. It is a sad commentary on our health care services that new units must be set up at least in part to accommodate some of the unhealthy symptoms in the health care system rather than to focus on the problem and rid the system of the "waiting disease" itself.

Most of us are aware of the psychosomatic nature of the disease process, yet the client has to add to that psychological trauma by being exposed to the frustrations of waiting. We give lip service to client-centered care, while the reality more closely resembles staff-centered care. We seek a therapeutic relationship and strive for the therapeutic use of self, yet fail to provide the mutual respect in the relationship upon which those concepts are based.

Employers are justified in complaining when scheduled appointments are not kept for their employees, who are allowed to be away from their job to attend to personal health problems. It is generally the employer who bears the cost of that time lost from the job. Consumer involvement and action may be the best solution to the problem of waiting.

The answer to the problem may not be as simple as one might expect. The wait may be an unconscious ploy whereby the mystique of the physician can be maintained. It may be a conscious or unconscious attempt to "psych out" the clients, i.e., the more painful the treatment, the more

[12]Walter L. Johnson and Leonard S. Rosenfeld, "Factors Affecting Waiting Time in Ambulatory Care Services," *Health Services Research,* Winter 1968, pp. 286–295.

effective the cure; the more bitter the pill, the better it works; the longer the wait, the more popular the doctor and the better the treatment. It may be a matter of attempts of health professionals to stay in control and perpetuate a one-upmanship between the consumer and the provider of care. While the wait does have message power, there may be many health care providers who are unaware of what it really communicates. The client is better informed than in the past and pays well for these services. Why then must he be treated as a second-class citizen? One clinic scheduled clients at 5-minute intervals. No one could possibly give any semblance of good care in that short period of time even if he did not consider the need to establish a relationship and do any client teaching.

The solution to the waiting room problem will not come overnight, but it will require the combined and continued efforts of consumers and providers alike. In the interim, health care workers should be ingenious in their use of the waiting time by doing health teaching and focusing on prevention of illness. Let us start an AWR (Abolish Waiting Rooms) Club and work for a better tomorrow in the hospitals, offices, and agencies where health care is given.

Whether it is the tempo or timing of a musical score, the rhythmic patterns of our biological processes, or the synchronization of the activities in our lives, duration and passing of time play a significant part in our intrapersonal and interpersonal communication. Whether we lay claim to and defend physical or professional territory, aggressive communication behavior is evident. The importance of the nonverbal spatial-temporal dimensions of communication cannot be denied even though much of this communication occurs out of awareness. There is even message value in the placement of the hands on clocks pictured in many newspaper advertisements. They are often placed at between 8:15 and 8:25, which is symbolic of the time of death of President Lincoln. We must continuously be conscious of the subtle and obvious message quality that comes from time and space, for they have far-reaching effects in human communication.

SUGGESTED BIBLIOGRAPHY

Allekian, Constance I.: "Intrusions of Territory and Personal Space: An Anxiety-Inducing Factor for Hospitalized Persons—An Exploratory Study," *Nursing Research*, **22** (3): 236–241, May–June 1973.

Fraisse, Paul: *The Psychology of Time*, Harper & Row, Publishers, New York, 1963.

Gibran, Kahlil: *The Prophet*, Alfred A. Knopf, Inc., New York, 1955.

Hall, Edward T.: *The Hidden Dimension*, Doubleday & Co., Inc., Garden City, N.Y., 1966.

Haythorn, William W. and Irwin Altman: "Together in Isolation," *Transaction*, **4:** 18–22, January–February 1967.

Husserl, Edmund: *The Phenomenology of Internal Time-Consciousness*, Indiana
    University Press, Bloomington, Ind., 1964.
McCroskey, James C.: *An Introduction to Rhetorical Communication*, 2d ed.,
    Prentice-Hall, Englewood Cliffs, N.J., 1972.
Moore, Wilbert E.: *Man, Time, and Society*, John Wiley & Sons, New York, 1963.
O'Neill, Nena and George O'Neill: *Open Marriage: A New Life Style for Couples*,
    J. B. Lippincott Co., Philadelphia, 1972.

Chapter 5

Interpersonal Communication

I must do these things in order to communicate: Become aware of you (discover you). Make you aware of me (uncover myself). Be ready to change during our conversation, and be willing to reveal my changes to you.

Hugh Prather

Most of our communication is interpersonal, involving two or more individuals sending, processing, and receiving messages. No social system can exist without communication among its members. Our ability to live and work alone, without communicating with others, is as futile as a one-handed clap.

We communicate in dyads, triads, and groups of varied size and type. The business world is filled with groups labeled "committees." Most interpersonal communication is conducted with only a few feet of distance between individuals in face-to-face contact. However, the interpersonal communication that is carried out through the mass media of radio and television also plays a prominent role in our lives. It is through our unique ability to use a variety of verbal and nonverbal symbols that we are able to communicate with even heterogeneous groups of people. Language is the universal code of communication for social interaction.

The foundation of all human communication is represented in the *intrapersonal* model. The *interpersonal* communication model is a composite of the number of intrapersonal models that corresponds to the number of persons in the encounter. The communication between a pair of individuals is the simplest form of interpersonal communication and was displayed in Figure 2-3. As the two intrapersonal models interact, the response of the sender (e.g., a word symbol) becomes a potential stimulus for the second individual. There are no passive roles in the interpersonal communication process. All of the individuals involved are actively processing information, and their roles are equally significant and responsible ones. Again, the overall goal is to match meaning, to obtain some agreement or close proximity in perceptions. Disagreements and dysfunctional communication do not come from value differences among individuals as much as from their differences in perception. In a mutually nonthreatening relationship, individuals' perceptions must be explored and clarified if effective communication between the individuals is to be realized. Generally the other fellow is not against us; he is basically egocentric and concerned with himself.

Try as we may, we cannot observe another's experience—we can never truly "get under the other fellow's skin" or "walk in his shoes." Empathic ability is a trait all of us possess but in varying degree. It is not easy to enter another's world and be sensitive to and able to judge another's feelings, attitudes, and behaviors. The difficulty in attaining empathic understanding is a limiting variable in our efforts to attain effective interpersonal communication. The important concept of empathy will be discussed in more detail in Chapter 9.

It is paradoxical that while *effective* interpersonal communication depends upon members in the interaction having similar world views, communication would not be necessary if all individuals in the group saw the same facts in the same way. There would be nothing to share if we all saw and felt alike. A degree of dissonance is required for communication to be needed.

Each individual in the encounter operates from his own unique frame of reference. The individuality of word-symbol meaning is clearly evident from the following story. John was walking downtown one day when he saw a penguin out in the middle of a busy intersection. He rushed out, picked up the penguin, and brought him over to the sidewalk. Just then an old friend came along and said, "John, what in the world are you doing with a penguin?" John said, "Well, he was in the middle of the street and I thought he would be hit by a car, so I picked him up, but I don't know what to do with him now." The friend suggested that John take the penguin to the zoo. John replied, "Gee, that's a great idea; I don't know why I didn't think of that," and went off down the street. The next day the friend spotted John walking down the street hand-in-flipper with the penguin and exclaimed, "I thought you were going to take that little fellow to the zoo!" John replied, "I did, and we had such a good time I am going to take him to the ballgame today." A simple example of dysfunctional communication where differences of word meaning between two individuals prevented the communication from being effective.

As we relate to others we expend considerable time and effort trying to make a good impression. In fact, a major obstacle in a first encounter is that we are so busy attempting to impress the other individual that we even fail to hear or remember his name. We accommodate to what we assume the other person expects of our actions and then wait for the reviews. The irony of it is that the other fellow is so preoccupied with trying to impress *us* that he is not attentive to us. A lot of testing is done in interpersonal relationships, especially during initial encounters. Group members test one another's boundaries of commitment, authority, intimacy, and expertise. Territorial governors are the socially acceptable constraints on groups as well as on individuals.

PURPOSE OF INTERPERSONAL COMMUNICATION

We spend much of our lives in group activities, in interpersonal communication, trying to solve problems, gain consensus, or accomplish some task. People organize themselves in groups to meet a need to relate to others through communication. Interpersonal communication makes society possible and affects the quality of life. Loneliness is a painful disease with no substitute except communication with others. Everybody needs somebody!

As a social animal, man interacts with others to meet both personal and social needs and gets to know himself and his effect upon others. We experience catharsis through the expression of our thoughts and feelings. Psychotherapeutic modalities are generally geared toward trying to persuade an individual to change his behavior and/or his associates to change their behavior in relation to him.

Interpersonal communication is carried out to influence others and move them towards or away from certain thoughts or actions. We can exert power; get support; and experience growth, pleasure, and meaning in life through self-expression and communication with others. The personal need to communicate is so great that Dial-A-Care projects are being sponsored by mental health organizations and churches across the country. The need for social intercourse is so great, particularly among the elderly, that some have been known to telephone the time bureau throughout the day just to hear someone's voice and at least temporarily alleviate their loneliness. Radio and television have been the salvation of many lonely individuals.

The service or therapy provided by the counselor, psychiatric nurse, or psychologist is accomplished through communication with the client. Much therapeutic communication takes place in the casual customer-barber, customer-beautician, and customer-bartender dyads. The customer may pay for the haircut, hairset, or drink but gets a lot of free counseling in addition.

It was Ardrey's contention that the territorial drive was the prime way, if not the exclusive means, by which man could meet his three basic needs simultaneously.[1] It is proposed here that all three basic needs can also be met through interpersonal communication. One's personality and *identity* are developed and maintained through communication with others in dyads and groups. The pleasure and excitement of interacting with others provides us with *stimulation*. It is stimulating to get and give information, to be creative as we engage others in problem solving, and to experience and facilitate change. Through interpersonal communication we influence, exert power, and gain *security* for ourselves. One feels more secure when one can coordinate one's expertise with others in group interaction and enhance one's purpose in life. Through communication with others, we can have identity rather than anonymity, stimulation rather than boredom, and security rather than the uncertainty often associated with individual rather than group effort.

SOME CHARACTERISTICS OF GROUPS

A group is any gathering of more than one person. Groups vary in their personnel makeup, size, and purpose; yet there are some basic factors that affect all group communication.

Type of Group

The pair, or *dyad*, is the least complex and most common group. The *triad*, or group consisting of three members, takes on added complexities. The additional member greatly affects the relationship established and the communication among its members. It is common to find in this triangulation that two members will take sides against the third. This is what frequently happens in families of three until the pattern is broken. A group of three is often the most difficult small group to deal with because there is always one individual on the outside and internal competition and jockeying for position is common. When the triad consists of three males, the

---

[1]Ardrey, *The Territorial Imperative*, pp. 336–337.

battle is for dominance, with the weakest one being excluded. Studies have shown that when the group is composed of three females, one is left out and the others make an effort to keep her in the group.

Intragroup communication involves members having a common goal and striving to attain group consensus. Some members facilitate group functioning while other are disruptive. If the group has no mutual goal, it may be more accurately referred to as a "bunch" or an "aggregate." Ineffective interaction and communication is readily evident from this collection of individuals because they have no mutual goals to give them a unified base of operation.

Intergroup communication is a linkage of related groups or a joint communication between two or more special interest groups to accomplish a common goal. Intergroup communication may be enhanced with a mediator or unbiased group facilitator giving direction and feedback to the groups as they function together.

Complex organizations and federal, state, and local government agencies are examples of *multigroups*. Communication is generally more formal than with intergroups. Multigroups frequently have rules and procedures to guide their behavior. Many diverse interests are represented, and competition is common.

Size of the Group

The type of group dictates in part the size of the group. Membership size is a critical variable in the interpersonal communication of the group. Each individual in the group represents one intrapersonal model of communication or communication unit. As membership size increases, there is a geometric increase in the interpersonal relationships, not a mere additive increase. There are not only an infinite number of dyadic communicative exchanges possible in each group but also varying combinations of interpersonal communication. The *nonadditive principle* operates, and each additional group member produces an increasingly complicated situation.[2] For example, a committee composed of 4 members has a possibility of 24 interactions. Tension generally develops when a committee numbers 6 because 720 possible interpersonal arrangements may occur. Groups of 8 members generally produce difficult relationships because of the potential interpersonal combinations, and muddled communication can be expected when the number reaches 12.

Group size is an important factor to consider whether the group is organized for the purpose of teaching, problem solving, or socializing. Effectiveness of interpersonal communication is generally inversely related to group size. Add to large group size the mixes of interactions and the

[2]Elwood Murray, Gerald M. Phillips, and J. David Truby, *Speech: Science-Art,* The Bobbs-Merrill Co., Indianapolis, Ind., 1969, pp. 199–200.

possibility of each member vying for leadership and power and attempting to be heard, and the problems are monumental.

Small Groups, which often number four to seven members, are the most common and generally the most effective ones for problem-solving tasks. Groups of small size may be more satisfying to the individuals involved because of greater opportunity to participate actively in the communication interchange. If the group is too large, there is a tendency for members to subgroup into one of more satisfying size. Most of the group research has been conducted on artificial laboratory groups. The practice of generalizing the findings to real groups with real problems that require solutions members must actually live with and put into practice must be questioned.

The *family* is the most common example of a small group. It has a style, patterns, and a communication network that dictate such behavior as who talks to whom and who clarifies the communication. Each family has it own cultural patterns of communication which must also be considered.

Life of the Group

An important factor in group communication is the life and history of the group. A *permanent* group is one with a past and a future. The family is a classic example. Permanent groups set up short- and long-range goals. A *temporary* group has great concern for the present but very little reference to the past or future, as one would of course expect. Temporary groups may be productive without a true sense of group belongingness or commitment being established. The level of trust established among group members depends upon the bonds and commitment to like goals and to other members. A higher level of trust and cohesiveness might be expected from the more permanent group, in which individuals have had time to test one another's motives and commitment.

Personality of the Group

The membership of the group is important to both the success of the task and the process or relationship. Humans are a part of the social enterprise, and personalities become synthesized into the process. No individual personalities are discretely identifiable in the group structure. Individual personalities as a collection do nothing to explain the characteristics of the group personality. We change and lose our previously unique and identifiable personality as we relate to others in a group. The total of the personalities of the members is more than and different from the sum of the personalities in the particular group. The situation is analogous to that of making a cake, where the milk, eggs, and flour are unidentifiable as individual ingredients when mixed together. The communication behavior of individuals and the group change with the addition or omission of a single member. A synergistic affect takes place.

Each group is unique in terms of the situation, environment, task, and, most of all, the individuals involved. Some members facilitate the group process, while others impede goal attainment through their verbal and nonverbal communication. Problems develop if there is great hetero-geneity among the members even though there may be a mutual purpose or goal. Any wonder government bureaucracies have difficulty accomplishing their tasks, when there is such heterogeneous membership on committees and each member attempts to foster his own self-interest! Individual and group identity are both strong. The personal identity "I" must not be lost, nor must it supersede the "we" of group activity.

There are a wide variety of characteristics of group and committee members. Some are said to be like mushrooms, keeping in the dark and out of sight and sound; others are like orchids, providing a nice centerpiece as they lend their status in the community and their prestige to the committee. Some members are like the potato—predictable and hard-working—while others are like the turnip, turning up at times of crisis but otherwise being dormant. Undoubtedly we all can identify individuals with whom we have worked in groups who fit these various characteristics.

The sensitivity of members to one another is reflected in the harmoni-ous relationship within the group and its ability to carry out its function. This characteristic is generally referred to as *empathic ability*. On the other hand, *dogmatism* displayed by group members may be regarded as one of the major limiting factors in interpersonal communication. We will always have varying degrees of open-mindedness and closed-mindedness in indi-viduals. More detailed discussion of both of these characteristics will be presented in subsequent chapters.

The Communication-Trust-Risk Paradigm

Communication, trust, and risk evolve as a paradigm or a construct in which each factor affects and is affected by each other in the interpersonal communication, as shown in Figure 5-1. The degree of interpersonal *trust* is an important variable that influences our communication and interaction with others. Trust paves the way to effective *communication* as individuals become more free and open in expressing their true and deep feelings and thoughts to others. Whether we first trust someone and that opens com-munication channels or we use communication behavior to establish a trusting relationship to further facilitate open communication, *risk* is involved. We risk that what we honestly say may be used against us or looked upon with disfavor by others. When we trust and disclose gut-level feelings, we are vulnerable and risk ridicule and rejection by others. We risk the hurt that comes from the psychological intimacy of personal trust.

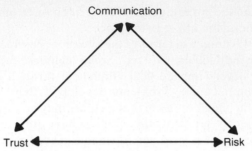

Figure 5-1   A paradigm in interpersonal communication.

There are many occasions in which we may be forced to trust someone and run the risk of being deceived by him because we need to release pent-up feelings. For example, in the client-counselor relationship individuals risk that they can trust the counselor not to reveal the honest feelings expressed because they need the therapeutic effect from that catharsis.

In building a trust relationship, game playing must stop and facades must be put aside. Following are the major factors that determine one's willingness to take the risk to trust others and communicate deep feelings:

1 *The trusting individual's personality.* Some individuals are basically more believing and trusting of others and more free and honest in communication with others. Those with this type of system might operate on the premise "Nothing ventured, nothing gained." The opposite and often pessimistic viewpoint would be "Nothing ventured, nothing lost."

2 *The particular individual being trusted.* Have you tested his trustworthiness in past situations? What is your past history with him? For example, how much would you be willing to risk and trust a statement made by former President Nixon, knowing his past? It hurts to risk when you think you have good odds, but it is foolhardy to risk and be hurt a second time. Once confidence is lost and belief destroyed, it is difficult to rebuild a climate of trust. One might be more willing to trust a friend, especially one who has been known for some time, rather than a stranger or a new acquaintance, other things being equal.

3 *The situation.* We may trust a person in one situation but not in another. This is often dependent upon what must be invested or risked versus the probability of benefits received. The situation also determines how important the benefits are to us. Distrust is most common when vested interests are involved. In some studies of mass media, it was found that a particular interest group distrusts and cannot accept what is being portrayed about *its* profession but thinks the media present an accurate portrayal of other professional groups. This finding may be a reflection of not being able to see ourselves as others see us or, if we do, wanting to deny it.

4 *Alternatives available*. Are there other choices and ones with less risk involved?

5 *Social and cultural factors*. Willingness to trust varies with our times. We have been deceived and our belief in people has been shattered by experiences and by what we have learned about government activities in recent years. We have become skeptical of the political process and less willing to trust our elected officials or be open to them in our communicative behaviors. At the same time, during the past decade and one-half increased members of training sessions and workshops have been conducted to encourage individuals to be risk takers and engage in self-disclosure.

In a climate of interpersonal trust, information sharing and better planning can be realized. A *consortium*, for example, is an assemblage of potential rivals or competitors who must become "men of goodwill" and put their collective interest above individual possessiveness of territory. The rewards are to maximize their impact through increased cooperation and to avoid duplication of effort. Growth can occur when a climate of mutual trust is established and communicated through shared information. Trust is the essential ingredient for developing effective consortiums or partnerships of peers.

One of the most serious crimes in interpersonal communication is violation of trust. The degree of trust between and among members of a group or organization is as good a predictor as any other of the effectiveness of communication within that group or organization. If individuals are willing to take the risk to trust and thus open communicative interchange or if, through open communication, a trusting atmosphere can be developed, effective communication is a true possibility.

The Individual Personality in the Relationship

While the group personality is not a summation of the personalities of its members, nor are discrete individual personalities identifiable in the interpersonal communication exchange, the personality of each member of the group does influence the relationship and the communication that results. The *Johari Window* conceptualized and labeled by Luft and Ingham in 1955 has been used extensively as a model of interpersonal behavior.[3] Each of the four quadrants of the window represents an area of one's personality that is known in varying degree to self and to others. Each of us has an *open or free area*, a *blind area*, a *hidden area*, and an *unknown or dark area* that significantly affect our interpersonal communication. The communication-trust-risk paradigm is related in various ways to each of the four areas.

The free or open area is information about self which is *known to self*

[3]Joseph Luft, *Of Human Interaction,* National Press Books, Palo Alto, Calif., 1969.

and to others. What are known are generally the more obvious and superficial aspects of one's personality and not the personal and intimate information about self. What is known might be such things as one's field of work, family composition, and likes and dislikes. Not much is risked in trusting others with this information. However, this also is information that is of least importance to our communication behavior with others. The situation in part dictates how open or free one is to reveal information about self. This area enlarges as trust is established and insight is gained.

The blind area includes information that is *unknown to self and known to others*. We cannot see our own house from inside, but others can see it. In the same way, others gather information about us from their perspective, to which we ourselves are blind. For example, we frequently have difficulty in recognizing our own voice on an audio tape yet can readily identify all of the other voices. We are strangers in the mirror: some part of self is out of our awareness yet known to others. The situation is analogous to the parable of Saint Luke 6:41 in the Bible, in which one is asked why he can see the mote or splinter in the other's eye but not see the beam or log in his own eye. What we do not know about ourselves *will* hurt us! Maybe *we* cannot tell when our feet smell, but others can. We often learn about our own traits, mannerisms, and behavior when others mimic us.

In this area of personality we need *feedback* from others to open our blind. The other person must risk telling us about ourselves and thereby possibly breaking our relationship. Many people cannot accept the findings from "seeing ourselves as others see us." We must also trust the other person and realize that he is not attacking our person with the feedback given, but rather directing us to see the behavior he perceives from us. The *Fishbowl* is an exercise used in group interaction. One task-oriented group, for example, is in an inner circle conducting its usual group activities, while a second group encircles the first and observes both group and individual behavior in the interaction. The second group then reports its perceptions to the inner group. The discussion serves to help the members of the inner group learn more about their group behavior and open their blind.

Individuals may learn about the behavior they exhibit by means of other simple games and exercises. One may use, for example, the simple question, "If you could come back into this world as a fish, fowl, animal, or bird, what would be your choice?" When exploring the possible reasons for their answers, individuals' personal needs, which are reflected in interpersonal behavior, become apparent. We may also have to risk the results of such experiences when participating in group exercises, for they may get to some of the more sensitive and deep areas of our personality and behavior.

The third quadrant of the Johari Window is the hidden area, which includes information *known to self but unknown to others*. Many of our communication problems result from misrepresenting self as we assume roles, play games, and wear masks. We put on a facade to hide certain vulnerable parts of self that we are unwilling to trust others to know about us. We hide much of our true self from others. Man is capable of *being* one thing and *seeming* to be someone different through his actions and verbal language. "Things are seldom what they seem; skim milk masquerades as cream."

We all have a tendency to keep important and personal data concealed from others, yet it is that very information that is crucial to interpersonal communication and understanding. Sometimes other individuals may be very perceptive and pick up subtle nonverbal cues that reveal the inner feelings we may be attempting to conceal from them. We monitor and censor our behavior and language in relation to what we *want* others to hear and believe about us and how much trust we have in them. Low self-disclosure makes it difficult to understand man's overt behavior and to communicate effectively.

Studies have revealed that very little disclosure occurs in most encounters. Individuals must feel safe to reveal what they know about themselves, and that requires trust in others. Being authentic, genuine, and open in our interpersonal behavior involves taking risks. The risks are greater as more intimate and deeper thoughts and feelings are expressed. When we hold back anger we are expressing a desire to preserve the relationship, even at the expense of destroying a part of self. Bottled-up emotions are just as difficult for all parties to deal with as verbalization and other overt expression of them.

Men typically are lower self-disclosers and reveal less personal information about themselves than women do. Too often we tell or reveal everything of what is really nothing and nothing of what is everything! While many facets of man and his personality are revealed as he trusts others and communicates with them, so many are hidden so that he may be safe. When under stress, we may remove our concealing mask and become painfully transparent. We may inadvertently be forced to disclose our thoughts and feelings. Psychotherapy is used to promote greater self-disclosure and authenticity on the part of the client. Many interpersonal training programs are directed toward helping individuals be more open and honest in their communication with others. Johnson[4] devoted an entire chapter to exercises aimed at facilitating self-disclosure.

The psychological climate must be conducive to feeling free to risk disclosure. Our cultural norms, customs, and social training dictate expectations relative to disclosure of self. They often force us to hide our true feelings from others and thus enlarge our hidden area and prevent us from

[4]David W. Johnson, *Reaching Out: Interpersonal Effectiveness and Self-Actualization,* Prentice-Hall, Englewood Cliffs, N.J., 1972, pp. 9–42.

being known to others. We fear being laughed at or shamed. Feelings of guilt, fear, and sorrow are often expressed in very devious ways that result in dysfunctional communication. Graffiti, which has been discussed previously, is one way to express deep feelings to others. One's identity is not known and therefore little is risked, but the communication from an "unknown" has little effect upon relationships. Intimacy in our communication with others does not have to be learned, just liberated. Social and other constraints that prevent the establishment of effective interpersonal communication must be eliminated.

The fourth quadrant is the unknown or dark area, which is *unknown to both self and others*. As William Ellery Channing said, "Every man is a volume if you know how to read him." Much of ourself is out of our awareness and is unknown to self as well as to others. As we go through life, we continuously become alert to cues that reveal some of self. If we would only take the time to explore some of the meaning behind our verbal utterances and overt behavior, we would reduce the size of the *unknown self* and better understand some of the reasons for problems in interpersonal communication. I do not like to swim and for many, many years had been deceiving myself by saying that it was because I fell into the water when I was 7 years old and have been fearful of water since that time. Upon taking myself to task and trying to identify that past experience, I found that I could not explain my fear on that basis. My thinking opened my unknown about myself, as I discovered that I obviously do not like to do anything I cannot do well, and swimming is one such activity. While this may appear to be an inconsequential discovery on the surface, it does have implications for my interpersonal communication in many areas. For example, I now realize how my motivation to do well, to excel in sports and the like, may not make relationships with me on the golf course, for example, very pleasurable for those who want to engage in a noncompetitive, leisurely activity.

We all need to continuously explore and question the reasons behind our relationships with others and gain new insights that will reduce the size of this dark area of our personality. We can get in touch with self as we disclose our feelings and thoughts to others. "How do I know what I think until I hear what I say?" speaks to this point. According to Jourard, "Every maladjusted person is a person who has not made himself known to another human being and in consequence does not know himself."[5] If we increase our awareness of our own communication behavior and others' responses to us, we can learn more about ourselves. A slip of the tongue, frequently labeled a *Freudian slip*, might reveal something of our behavior if we would attend to it and study it. Books are available which provide

[5]Sidney M. Jourard, *The Transparent Self*, D. Van Nostrand Co., Princeton, N.J., 1964, p. 26.

communication exercises for experiential learning in dyads and groups to help one learn about self. Books by Johnson[6] and by O'Banion and O'Connell[7] are examples.

The four areas of one's personality reflect the known and unknown about the individuals in relationship with one another. The communication trust-risk paradigm is in juxtaposition with each quadrant in varying degrees. When we trust and thereby risk self-disclosure in interpersonal encounters, we are indeed vulnerable. However, if effective interpersonal communication is our aim, we must be authentic and open in our relationship with others. Dysfunctional communication is inevitable if our *free* area is small while the *blind, hidden,* and *dark* areas of our personality are disproportionately large.

METHODOLOGIES FOR GROUP RESEARCH

There are many research instruments available for the study of various aspects of group behavior and interpersonal communication. A few of the more commonly used ones include process recording, Bales's Interaction Process Analysis, sociometry, FIRO-B, sociodrama, and sculpting. The results of a monumental task of categorizing and presenting in summary form the findings from the wealth of small-group-behavior research appear in the book entitled *Small Group Research*.[8] It is suggested as a reference to provide the reader with some idea of the direction and extent of the interpersonal research that has been conducted.

Process Recording and Analysis

Process recording has been used extensively as a teaching tool in the areas of psychiatry and psychiatric nursing. It involves the recording of the verbal and nonverbal behavior exhibited in the interaction by one of the group participants. The recording is made *after* the interaction and is used to reflect on what actually took place between the individuals involved. Interpretation and analysis are made and used as a basis for learning and for future encounters.

Bales's Interaction Process Analysis (IPA)[9]

The IPA tool was developed to study interactions by making formal observations and analyses of the interactions. It is a recording and tabula-

[6]Johnson, *Reaching Out.*
[7]Terry O'Banion and April O'Connell, *The Shared Journey: An Introduction to Encounter,* Prentice-Hall, Englewood Cliffs, N.J., 1970.
[8]Joseph E. McGrath and Irwin Altman, *Small Group Research,* Holt, Rinehart and Winston, New York, 1966.
[9]Robert F. Bales, *Interaction Process Analysis,* Addison-Wesley Publishing Co., Inc., Reading, Mass., 1950.

tion of utterances that relate to the relationship, or *process*, and to the *task* of the group. One or more nonparticipant observers systematically record the interaction of members in a small group through a one-way mirror. Nonverbal communication is also observed and recorded. At 15-minute intervals during the group interaction, communication is classified for each group member into the appropriate one of 12 categories.[10] The categories include such activities as giving and repeating information, clarifying and confirming others, giving opinion, evaluating, analyzing, and expressing feelings. The tabulation also identifies whether the communication was positive or negative. Bales's IPA instrument provides information on high, low, and intermediate interactors in the group and identifies the functions each member seems to play in the interpersonal exchange.

Sociometry

The well-known psychiatrist Dr. J.L. Moreno introduced sociometry in 1931 as a means of obtaining a quantitative measure of interpersonal phenomena. Sociometry is prescriptive as well as descriptive in nature. It provides a means for restructuring groups for more effective functioning as well as showing the attraction and repulsion of members in a given group, which may explain some of the interpersonal behavior and communication of the group.

The sociometric test provides valuable empirical data relating to a person's perception of his social environment. The test is a simple request: "If you were on a committee, list, in order of preference, the persons *from this group* you would most like to have on your committee" or "List in order of choice those *from this group* whom you would most like to be with socially." Generally first, second, and third choices are asked to be identified. Choices are tabulated for each group member, and an arbitrary numerical value is assigned to first, second, and third choices. For example, first choice may carry a 3-point value, second choice may be assigned 2 points, and third choice may receive 1 point. The total choice values for each member are placed in rank order, and through the use of a graph one identifies the most and least chosen members of the group for each specific activity, e.g., committee work or social activity, as shown in Figure 5-2. Sociometric choice depends heavily on the work or activity for which the membership choice is being made. Seldom will individuals attain the same choice value for different activities. However, in Figure 5-2, subject A did rank first in both committee work and social activity and even scored similar total point values (21 to 23 points) on both activities. These findings were obtained from an actual 21-member group. While anonymity must be

---

[10]Robert F. Bales, "How People Interact in Conferences," in Alfred G. Smith (ed.) *Communication and Culture*, Holt, Rinehart and Winston, New York, 1966, pp. 94–102.

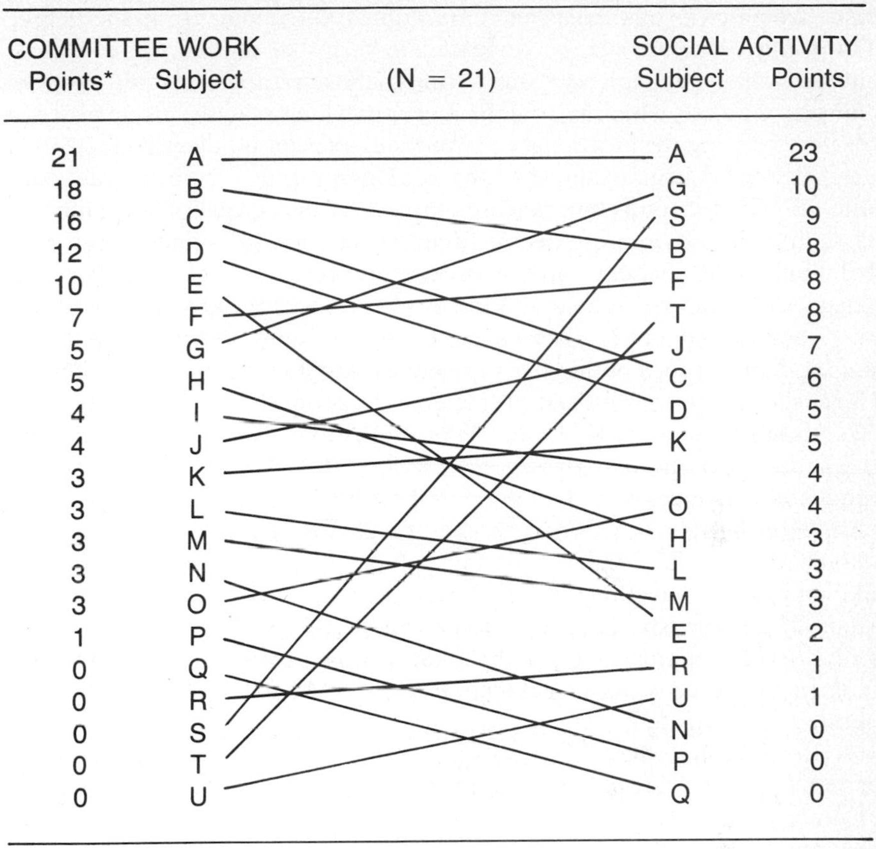

COMMITTEE WORK		(N = 21)	SOCIAL ACTIVITY	
Points*	Subject		Subject	Points
21	A		A	23
18	B		G	10
16	C		S	9
12	D		B	8
10	E		F	8
7	F		T	8
5	G		J	7
5	H		C	6
4	I		D	5
4	J		K	5
3	K		I	4
3	L		O	4
3	M		H	3
3	N		L	3
3	O		M	3
1	P		E	2
0	Q		R	1
0	R		U	1
0	S		N	0
0	T		P	0
0	U		Q	0

*1st choice = 3 points
 2nd choice = 2 points
 3rd choice = 1 point

Figure 5-2 Rank order of choices of group members for committee work compared with social activity.

assured when administering the test, personality qualities and communication skill of subject A would prove an interesting study. Subjects R, F, and K changed their ranking position only one rank. For social activity subject E dropped 10 ranks below her committee-work ranking. Subject S made the greatest change in ranked choice. She moved up from the third *least* chosen for committee work to the third *most* chosen for social activity. All other members changed their rank either up or down from their committee-work rank in varying degrees.

The *sociogram* is the form used to display the raw data obtained from sociometric testing of choices. A pictorial display of choices allows one to visualize patterns of choices and communication among group members. The group structure can be reviewed in terms of mutual or reciprocal choices, chains of choices, "stars" (most chosen), and "isolates" (never chosen). Cliques, which may be the disruptive factors in the group process that are causing dysfunctional communication, can be identified.

Figure 5-3 is an example of the sociogram drawn from the raw data when first and second choices were obtained from a group of 20 members. If all first choices, represented in Figure 5-3 by the solid line, are given a point value of 2, and all second choices, represented by the broken line, are assigned a value of 1, subject P is the obvious star of the group, with a total of 17 points. Subject N places second but far below P, with a total of 6 points. Some groups of this size may have a number of stars. More can be learned about this group and projected interaction by further study.

Individuals B, E, K, L, and R are all isolates—no one has selected them as either his first or second choice. If a third choice had been requested, chances are that the number of isolates would have been reduced. The star (P) was first choice of eight group members and second choice of one. The number of mutual or reciprocal choices between members tells something about the cohesiveness of the group. In this study, there were six reciprocal choices made (J-P, S-M, G-O, O-M, N-H, and T-P). The mutual selection by J and P was the only instance in which both reciprocated with a first choice. P, O, and M had both first and second choices reciprocated.

In addition to the sociogram's providing a pictorial description of the group, it also provides clues as to how members of the large group might be structured into effectively functioning smaller groups. Studies have shown that any individual's performance is at its best when he is working with a partner of his own choosing. Performance has been found to be superior even to that of individuals who have made reciprocal choices. Isolates are often placed with the overchosen in hopes of helping them develop their capabilities. In the group interaction displayed in Figure 5-3, the strong single star (P) might be placed in a smaller group with some of the identified isolates. Five isolates in a group of 20 might be indicative of the difficulty often experienced when the size of the group is so large that it restricts involvement of all members. Subjects B, E, and R, who chose P as their first choice, might be more active if placed in a group with the star. Regrouping after a study of sociometric choices has also been helpful in identifying and evaluating the leadership role. If the original group of 20 had been regrouped into three smaller groups of 6 or 7 members, one would expect to find improved interpersonal communication. After the members of the three small groups had worked together and gotten to know each other, another sociometric test with a sociogram drawn to describe interactional patterns that had developed would have been in order.

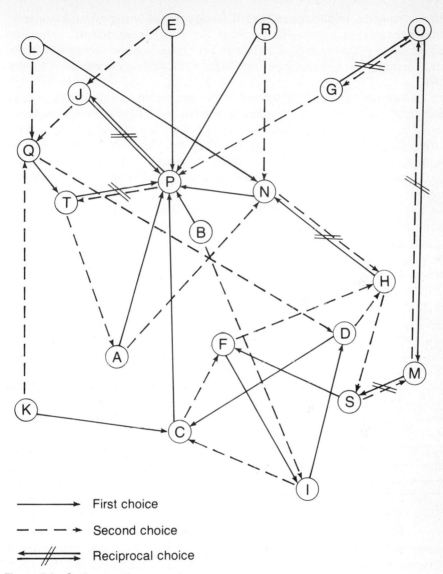

First choice

- - - → Second choice

Reciprocal choice

Figure 5-3 Sociogram of sociometric choices.

FIRO-B

Sociometry reveals our interpersonal attraction to others but says nothing about the reason for the choices that are made. While restructuring groups for more effective interpersonal behavior is possible without knowing the reason for the choices, there are situations in which the reason for the choice may be important. FIRO-B (fundamental interpersonal orientation–behavior) is a three-dimensional theory of interpersonal behavior developed by Schutz.[11] The FIRO-B Test based on the theory has been used in many ways, including efforts to get compatability in group composition.

Everyone orients self toward other people in characteristic ways. Schutz theorized that people need people for three kinds of relationships: *inclusion, control,* and *affection* (ICA). We may *express* these needs toward others and/or there may be ways in which we *want* others to behave toward us. People obviously differ greatly in what they first look for in others. The test responses for each individual are matched to obtain compatible group composition.

It seemed feasible that if the sociometric test could reveal interpersonal choices and the FIRO-B test would give the reason for the choices, a study using the combined findings from these two instruments would provide some important answers relative to group interaction. A study was designed and conducted using 73 professional nurse subjects who were employed in the area of nursing administration and were participants in the last of a series of leadership workshops.[12] The findings revealed that there was no significant difference between the "most chosen" and "never chosen" as revealed by the sociometric test for either expressed or wanted behavior on the inclusion and control dimensions as tested with the FIRO-B instrument. However, there was a significant difference at the 1 percent level of confidence for both expressed and wanted behavior for the affection dimension. The selection of group membership could then be made only on the basis of expressed and wanted affection. It may be significant that all but one of the 73 subjects were women. The findings might corroborate findings from other studies which showed that women tend to look for personality traits and social techniques while men are most interested in status and achievement factors in choosing group members.

Sociodrama

The sociodrama is a type of role play or acting out of a social issue or case study in an effort to improve group behavior. It is the spontaneous enactment of social situations and results in experiential learning. It consists of four steps: (1) the idea, (2) the warmup, where some very basic questions are proposed to help the actors get into the mood of the situation, (3) enactment through one or more scenes, and (4) discussion or catharsis, in which the actors' feelings are explored.

[11]William C. Schutz, *FIRO: A Three-Dimensional Theory of Interpersonal Behavior,* Holt, Rinehart and Winston, New York, 1960.
[12]Margaret L. Pluckhan, "An Investigation of Sociometric Choices in Various Behavioral Settings," *Handbook of International Sociometry,* **VII**: 43–51, 1973.

Sociodrama is similar to psychodrama except that it is an acting out of a dramatic presentation of a social problem involving members of a group. Psychodrama focuses more on dramatizing individual behavior.

Sculpting

Sculpting is yet another means of studying group interaction and helping individual members and groups gain insight into their interpersonal behavior. This technique is often used with families. Family members describe their relationship to one another by the way they arrange their bodies in space at a particular point in time. For example, a family member may be asked to describe his family of origin by placing group members in representative relationship to one another. Furniture and other objects may be used to represent missing members and other factors that help describe family relationships.

The experience is primarily nonverbal. The use of the verbal language is de-emphasized. The nonverbal description is found to be more helpful in having group members gain insight and reorganize their perceptions than are verbal utterances. Verbal discussion follows the nonverbal discourse in an effort to increase understanding of the family dynamics.

Simon described sculpting as "the plastic representation of unconscious themes."[13] He found that adolescents are usually excellent sculptors because of both their insight into family truths and their view of the task as a way of manipulating their elders.

Sculpting is used for diagnostic purposes as well as an adjunct to other forms of family therapy. The pictorial representation of family relationships by various family members often points out incongruent realities among its members. These discrepancies may be the primary factors that cause dysfunctional communication within the family unit. Sculpting bears some resemblance to psychodrama and sociodrama but uses more nonverbal than verbal techniques.

MASS MEDIA

While the mass media are primarily the concern of the field of communications technology, they are a powerful form of interpersonal communication and therefore warrant some mention in this text on human communication. The mass media have been labeled "the extensions of man" by McLuhan.[14] Certainly our world has outgrown the reach of the voice and there are no geographical limits to our interpersonal communication. Rapid

---

[13]Robert M. Simon, "Sculpting the Family," *Family Process,* 11(1): 51, March 1972.
[14]Marshall McLuhan, *Understanding Media: The Extensions of Man,* McGraw-Hill Book Co., New York, 1964.

advances in communications technology during the past two decades in particular have extended our interpersonal boundaries. Messages have been sent and received from outer space, from the moon and from Mars.

Television in particular, whose messages hit both our auditory and visual sense organs, has had a significant impact on our lives. Audiovisual as well as printed messages from around the world have brought the confines of the world into our living room through sophisticated telecommunications equipment. This worldwide physical togetherness has laid the groundwork for cooperative research and more rapid and extensive dissemination of findings for the benefit of all mankind.

Television is a social instrument that makes the audience a vicarious participant even though, as with the written message, immediate feedback may be given but not be accessible to the media message senders. Viewers identify with the characters in the TV soap operas and feel their experience as though the viewers had had the experience in real life. This vicarious experience is referred to as *anticipatory socialization*, and what is learned can be applied to real-life interpersonal encounters. A television viewer may experience the role of the client, for example, as he watches any number of the hospital-centered programs, before he actually enters that role. If the media present a false image of the client role, the health care setting, or individuals providing health care, they have done a disservice to the consumer and provider of that care. This is one of the reasons health care providers have insisted on monitoring and reviewing what is to be presented to the potential consumer of their services.

The mass media have stimulated and nourished a mass culture. They provide entertainment, education, and culture. They have lifted our horizons and created a world view that would not be possible just by means of face-to-face relationships. Television can fit a 60-piece orchestra into our living room and provide the experiences that many people could otherwise never afford or have. Telecommunications technology is already playing an important role in the delivery of health care, especially through satellite clinics in the rural areas of our country. Citizen band radios opened interpersonal communication with virtual strangers and saved lives and time in addition.

Franklin Delano Roosevelt was the first President to make full use of the radio. His popular "fireside chats" brought him into interpersonal communication with all Americans. The radio had become a healthy rival to the newspaper media. Since that time, television has played an influential role in presidential elections and has even been accused of altering the results of the elections following the famous Kennedy-Nixon debates. More than has the hard-cover book, the paperback book has provided interpersonal experiences through written communication. Seldom is an individual seen to board a commercial airplane without a paperback book tucked in a briefcase, purse, or coat pocket.

Many questions have been raised regarding both the beneficial and the detrimental effects of the mass media, television in particular, upon our way of life and the family unit. Many of the positive effects have already been discussed. In terms of the negative effects, the technologies have been accused of creating an unhealthy and violent environment. There is no question of the mass media exerting widespread influence and power in our society. Television has been accused of producing a passivity-fantasy-escape syndrome that is producing social problems. Some people claim that we are becoming an impersonalized society as even our education comes via the television tube and no immediate feedback or interchange is possible.

Findings of research into the effects of television on human behavior have been less than conclusive due to a lack of research tools available. Special monitors have been randomly placed on TV sets in homes across the country to assess viewing preferences as well as to answer questions regarding effects on behavior. However, it is not enough to know that the TV set is turned on and to a particular program, for this reveals nothing about whether individuals are actually watching the program and which members of the family are watching, let alone the psychological effect it has on them.

Those working with the mass media support their obviously biased opinion that *influence* exists, as it does in all forms of interpersonal communication, in the direction the viewer himself wants to go. Any ill effects are therefore blamed on the viewers themselves. The researchers claim that communication is not merely a pouring in and receiving of information, and therefore one cannot equate exposure with effect or stimulus with response. They claim that the external forces may monitor but the internal forces dictate. Efforts have been made to write laws to regulate television programming, but without research findings to support the belief that psychic and social disturbances are related to our mass media, little can be done in the way of regulation and control.

SUGGESTED BIBLIOGRAPHY

Ardery, Robert: *The Territorial Imperative*, Atheneum Publishers, New York, 1966.

Beinstein, Judith, "Conversation in Public Places," *Journal of Communication*, **25**(1):85–95, Winter 1975.

Berne, Eric: *Games People Play: The Psychology of Human Relationships*, Grove Press, New York, 1964.

Brooks, William D. and Philip Emmert: *Interpersonal Communication*, Wm. C. Brown Co., Publishers, Dubuque, Iowa, 1976.

Brown, Barbara B: *New Mind, New Body: Bio-feedback: New Directions for the Mind*, Harper and Row, Publishers, New York, 1974.

Etzioni, Amitai, Kenneth Laudon, and Sara Lipson: "Participatory Technology: The Minerva Communications Tree," *Journal of Communication*, **25**(2):64–74, Spring 1975.

Giffin, Kim and Bobby R. Patton: *Fundamentals of Interpersonal Communication*, Harper & Row, Publishers, New York, 1971.

Hare, A. Paul, Edgar F. Borgatta, and Robert F. Bales (eds.): *Small Groups: Studies in Social Interaction*, rev. ed., Alfred Knopf, New York, 1965.

Howe, Reuel L.: *The Miracle of Dialogue*, The Seabury Press, New York, 1963.

Johnson, David W.: *Reaching Out: Interpersonal Effectiveness and Self-Actualization*, Prentice-Hall, Inc., Englewood Cliffs, N.J., 1972.

Jourard, Sidney M.: *The Transparent Self*, D. Van Nostrand Co., Princeton, N.J., 1964.

Karlins, Marvin and Lewis M. Andrews: *Biofeedback: Turning on the Power of Your Mind*, J.B. Lippincott Co., Philadelphia, 1972.

Miller, Gerald R. and Mark Steinberg: *Between People: A New Analysis of Interpersonal Communication*, Science Research Associates, Chicago, Ill., 1975.

Miller, Neal E., David Shapiro, and John Stoyva (eds.): *Biofeedback and Self-Control*, Aldine-Atherton, New York, 1971.

Moreno, J. L. (ed.): *The Sociometry Reader*, The Free Press of Glencoe, New York, 1960.

Pluckhan, Margaret L.: "An Investigation of Sociometric Choices in Various Behavioral Settings," *Handbook of International Sociometry*, **VII**, 1973.

Chapter 6

The Interpersonal
Communication Contract

*Most controversies would soon be ended, if those engaged in them would first
accurately define their terms, and then adhere to their definitions.*

Tyron Edwards

We have already discussed a semblance of a contract—one that an individual makes with himself. The filtering and symbolic transformation process identified in the intrapersonal communication model is a reflection of the personal contract to maintain a degree of internal consistency and harmony between the programmed data stored in one's memory bank and new inputs from the external world.

An equally important contract is the one that is a part of all interpersonal communication encounters. The *communication contract* is a binding agreement among two or more persons which dictates the modus operandi, or rules and procedures to be followed by them, as they communicate with one another. While most individuals may not have labeled their "rules of encounter" a *"contract"* or identified a particular breakdown in communication as a "breach of contract," their inner feelings and overt expressions are a reflection of it nonetheless. In fact, one is often not aware of the existence of rules or specific terms of the contract until they have been broken.

Few authors have focused attention on the interpersonal communication contract per se. However, this author is of the opinion that the contract bears so heavily on the goal of effective interpersonal communication that there is ample justification for devoting an entire chapter to the subject. All individuals and their relationship to one another are affected by the contract and must therefore be aware of it and its effects.

IMPLIED AND EXPLICIT CONTRACTS

The contract may be implied or explicit, but the consequences of breaking either type are equally devitalizing to the communication process. Most of our daily business and social interpersonal communication operates with an *implied* contract by which general assumptions and expectations are habitually applied to our interpersonal symbolic commitments. The rules are in the minds of the group members and represent the expected behavior of the members. It is not surprising that terms of an implied contract are often broken when each individual member draws up his own rules of procedure, which are neither known nor accepted by other members. Some of the rules have been socially and culturally established while others are derived from our personal value and belief systems.

The *explicit* communication contract has terms that are spelled out, externally visible, and definite. Members in the social interaction are all aware of them even though all may not have been equally involved in their formulation and acceptance. The explicit contract is void of the vagueness and ambiguity present with an implied contract. An example of an explicit contract is a brochure advertising a conference or a printed program of a continuing education workshop. While an explicit contract may tend to formalize an interpersonal relationship, the potential for developing communication problems is generally reduced when group members are aware of the rules governing their social interaction. Parlimentary rules and Robert's Rules of Order are examples of very formal explicit interpersonal communication contracts that are set up to guide group members' behavior. Specific rules are set up for addressing the chair, making formal motions, seconding the motion, and asking for a majority or consensus vote on an issue. An individual with expertise in parlimentary procedure is frequently employed to interpret the rules to members at professional meetings and conventions. The degree of formality of an event or situation dictates the limits to spontaneous interaction among group members.

All members of the social interaction share in the responsibility to fulfill the contract commitments. Abiding by the terms of the contract enhances the possibility of successful completion of the group task as well as the maintenance of a harmonious group relationship. Participants vary in their ability to tolerate members who break the rules of the contract. An individual may be excused for failing to behave in the expected way a first time, especially if the group was operating under an implied contract, but a second breach of contract may result in dysfunctional communication in the group. There is a tendency to alienate oneself from individuals and from further exchanges with them if the contractual agreement is not kept.

Cross-cultural variation in expectations and assumptions must also be recognized. Rules of interpersonal communication become generally accepted by a particular culture. For example, if one attends a lecture, it is generally expected that members of the audience will have little, if any, opportunity to engage in verbal exchange with the speaker unless that option is explicitly announced. The game of bridge is essentially a game of interpersonal contracts. Symbols are used to bid a hand, and responses from one's partner are expected to follow some preestablished rules. Cross-cultural problems with assumptions about rules are analogous to the situation in which the bridge player bids a "short club" to a partner who is not familiar with the meaning of that bid, the partner reads it as a conventional club bid, and their interpersonal relationship as well as their score may suffer.

Some individuals try to avoid the explicit contract and have the freedom that an implied contract allows. Groups may be forced to go from an implied to an explicit contract when communication becomes so pathological that the group no longer can function. All social interaction behavior must then be renegotiated.

TERMS OF THE CONTRACT

Whether the social interaction or interpersonal communication is between the author of a book and its readers or a lecturer and his audience or among members of a group or committee, there are expectations and assumptions about the behavior of the individuals involved which enter into the implied or explicit contractual agreement. Behavior is directed toward an assumed or explicit purpose of the interaction, which in turn dictates the content and title, where appropriate. Communication rules are made in terms of the psychological climate expected and the relationship among group members. The verbal language and spatial and temporal aspects of communication are also designated in the terms of the contract. The setting or situation carries some preconceived notions of the interpersonal communication behavior that is appropriate and expected. Finally, members have expectations relative to rewards from the social encounter.

Purpose

One would be ill-advised to assume that because a committee has been formed, any or all of the members know of its overall *purpose* as well as the specific objective of a particular session. While interpersonal communication has a basic purpose of influencing, there are more definitive reasons why people group themselves and engage in social interactions. The purpose might be to exchange points of view or information, to creatively explore new ways to provide a service, to solve a particular problem, or just to socialize. Whatever the purpose, all members must direct their communication behavior toward that goal. How often have you been in a meeting in which everyone was "spinning his wheels" and the group was becoming frustrated and irritated with the lack of progress being made? Finally, when someone was bold enough to ask what the purpose of the meeting was to be, it became readily apparent that there was no agreement among the group members as to purpose in terms of the implied contract under which they had been operating.

Content and Title

The *content* or focus of the discussion would be expected to be in accord with the purpose of the group encounter. Without some explicit rules or guidelines and mutually accepted purpose, individuals might tend to deviate from the focus of the discussion. A *title*, which often accompanies interpersonal communication activities such as a lecture, conference, book, article, or committee, should be expected to be in concert with the content around which the interpersonal communication behavior will be directed. Authors and conference leaders in particular do a disservice to their readers and audience when they use short colloquial titles that do not reflect the content. Just as you cannot tell a book by its cover, so you often cannot expect the content to be reflected in the title. It seems to be a popular practice for a title to consist of a simple word, followed by a colon and words that more clearly reflect the content of the book. The book by Schutz entitled *Joy: Expanding Human Awareness*[1] or Watts's *The Book: On the Taboo against Knowing Who You are*[2] are examples.

It is generally assumed that when a course is called a "seminar," all members of that interpersonal experience, including the instructor, will have equal chance to express their ideas. If the instructor places himself in front of the room, apart from the students, and lectures to them, there is a breach of contract. Even if the instructor stays in close spatial relationship

---

[1]William C. Schutz, *Joy: Expanding Human Awareness,* Grove Press, New York, 1967.

[2]Alan W. Watts, *The Book: On the Taboo against Knowing Who You Are,* Collier Books, New York, 1966.

with the students, indicative of seminar-type discussion, but monopolizes the conversation, it likely is viewed as a violation of the communication agreement.

When the interaction is labeled a "panel," by convention this implies that each panel member will be assigned a limited period of time to present his case, then there will be an interchange among panel members directed by the moderator. The moderator, by implication, will not engage in any discourse other than a possible summary of the session. The moderator will call upon the audience for their inputs. If the moderator does not explicitly define the rules of the game to be followed, the generally accepted patterns of communication for a panel are implied. A "lecture" implies that the majority of the verbalization will come from the lecturer and the audience will participate verbally only if explicitly directed.

A "workshop" generally implies that the participants will be active and engage in experiential learning sessions. In the years when T-groups and sensitivity training were in vogue, participant involvement was often rather secretly thrust on the audience and caused hostility, for it was viewed as a breach of contract, especially when the title was a misnomer. Few of us have not felt cheated at some time or another when attending a lecture under a title that in no way reflected the content that was presented. One lecture entitled "Dialectical Tensions" ended up being a discussion of research. Midway through the lecture, the speaker admitted that he had changed the topic under contract, but he still broke the contract under which the audience had entered into interpersonal exchange with him. Obviously the rewards that had been expected by the audience were not received. Another example of breaking terms of a contract was a speech entitled "Social Problems Involving the Medical Care Team." The doctor talked exclusively about his own personal experiences in dealing with dying patients. The topic came across as more of a catharsis for the doctor than information for the audience. If members of a group fail to perceive congruence between the explicit title and the content and basic purpose of the interpersonal communication, breakdown in communication can be expected.

Psychological Climate

While we all know that there are thoughts and feelings we disguise from others, for the most part we function in relationship with others on the premise that what is being said is reliable and there is no phoniness in the encounter. Yet there are always those who suspect a hidden agenda and take what is being said with reservation. We communicate in terms of the way we perceive the members in relationship to one another and the implied rules *we* have set down. If we perceive a healthy group climate, we may have the implied rule that we will confront members whose verbal statements we question. It will generally be expected that a designated leader will have a priviledged position in the exchange. Rules regarding giving and receiving feedback and acceptable strategies for helping members see the point of view of others may have to be clarified early in the encounter and possibly become explicit terms of the contract. Establishing and maintaining a group climate that fosters effective interpersonal communication rests heavily on the terms of the implied or explicit contract.

Relationship of Members

There are two major dichotomies regarding the relationship of members to one another which enter into the interpersonal communication contract. Individuals contract for and communicate on the basis of either a dialogical or a monological relationship and either a symmetrical or a complementary relationship with members of the group.

Dialogical or Monological Relationship   A *dialogue* is one in which members are free to reveal self and accept the revelation of others. There is a mutualism, equality, and authenticity to the relationship. A *monologue*, conversely, is characterized by self-centeredness of members, who view other members as being there to serve them. It is largely a closed system, in which individuals are not open to inputs from others. This type of relationship fosters alienation and psychological distance among members, while the dialogical relationship tends to bring members together. Marked differences in the terms of the contract and the interpersonal communication patterns of the group will be evident whether the individuals perceive a dialogical or a monological relationship.

Symmetrical or Complementary Relationship   It is generally expected that there will be varying degree of participation by members of a group. One may or may not expect there to be some hierarchical structuring or pecking order in the communication behavior of group members. If members are perceived as equals, a *symmetrical* relationship exists and the communication behavior of all members is expected to be similar. A social gathering or a conversation between friends might most clearly exemplify a symmetrical relationship. The purpose and focus of the conversation, as well as the perceived expertise of the group members relative to it, influence the way the relationship is perceived and the terms of the contract.

Different types of communication behavior are evident if the relationship is perceived as *complementary*. Some members are superior to others, and a hierarchical structuring is made evident by the varied communication behavior exhibited by the members. This type of relationship is the lecturer-audience, teacher-student, parent-child, counselor-client, or doctor-patient relationship. One member may give advice; the other may take it. Authority and control are factors in the relationship. A parent may be in control and exhibit behavior to reflect that power. However, as the child grows to adulthood, a more symmetrical relationship and its associated communication patterns may develop. Some parent-child conflicts result when the child no longer views his role as a subservient one. Dysfunctional communication results when members of a dyad develop a contract based on different perceptions of their relationship to one another.

Communication patterns vary greatly from family to family, depending upon how the relationship among its members is perceived by each of them. Frequently complementary relationships are operating, under which parental rules govern the communication patterns and children are given little opportunity to serve as equals in decision making. It would be interesting to study married couples to determine how each member of the pair perceives the relationship. If one member is perceived as being in a subservient role, their communication and marriage may be more inclined to result in problems than if a symmetrical relationship is perceived by both members and serves as a part of their communication contract. Couples communicate as each perceives the relationship and the rules related to it.

Verbal Language

Members of an English-speaking group would feel that the terms of the implied contract had been broken if the encounter were not conducted in English, unless, of course, some rules to the contrary had been explicitly pointed out. The same rules might be implied relative to the use of *jargon*. Unless all group members are familiar with a particular terminology of a discipline, one does not expect it to be used.

A breach of an implied contract might also be assumed if a group member was left out of the discussion because of the *vocabulary* that was used. When entering into a contract, one generally expects that the level of comprehension of the language will fit the audience or group. The terms of the contract appear to be broken if either the vocabulary used tends to be above one's comprehension or one feels that others are talking down to him. Flesch was concerned that the verbal language fit the audience and popularized the concept of *readability*. He developed a tool to determine readability and set up norms based on sentence length in words, word length in syllables, percentage of personal words, and percentage of personal sentences.[3] Possibly some of the hostility associated with completing the complex federal income tax forms is due to the fact that while they must be completed by individuals of varying education and intellectual backgrounds, they can be barely understood by even more educated

[3]Rudolf Flesch, *The Art of Readable Writing*, Collier-Macmillan, London, 1949, pp. 226–230.

individuals. Lawyers and accountants have become wealthy due to that fact.

The *speed and volume* of a person's verbal utterances are also factors to consider. An individual may sense a break in their implied contract if he cannot comprehend what is being said either because the other person(s) are talking much too rapidly or not loud enough to be heard. A common negative evaluation of a conference is that the participants could not hear the speaker. The frustration is analogous to that of the reader who misses words and thoughts because the binding on a book has obliterated some of the words.

A generally accepted implied rule of interpersonal communication is that individuals will share the speaking time and *take turns talking*. Interrupting others when they are talking or *talking when others are talking* generally calls forth hostile behavior. Locke said, "There cannot be a greater rudeness than to interrupt another in the current of his discourse." Another generally assumed rule is that when individuals are not speaking, they will be *attentive* to those who are speaking.

Spatial and Temporal Aspects

Some rules of interpersonal communication behavior are implied from the *spatial* relationship among members, the seating arrangement, and the size of the group. Tradition generally dictates that when individuals are seated around a rectangular table, the person occupying the "head of the table" has greater influence and power than the others. The person seated in a high-backed chair or behind a desk often is viewed as one with some regal status. That perception carries with it expectations and rules regarding his communication behavior.

A pleasant breach of contract may occur when a speaker broaches the public space or physical distance nonverbally by bringing the audience into social and possibly personal space through verbal sharing of some intimate experience or making fun of himself. Group members may be irritated if they expected that there would be privacy to their space, yet phone calls and other noise factors interrupt their encounter.

The explicit "*time* contract" associated with clinic appointments was presented in Chapter 4. Hostile reactions to breaking of the time contract may be more pronounced when it is explicit than when it is an implied part of the contract. Time-oriented individuals may allow no excuse for breaking time limits. The time allowed for each person to speak depends in part upon the size of the group and rules regarding time sharing. If the relationship is considered to be symmetrical, implied rules may legislate equal time for each group member. In London a committee recommended that time clocks be installed in the House of Lords to monitor speeches. A sponsor of the recommendation said that no time limit would be set for speeches but that each speaker would be able to see two or more clocks—the idea being that all men of high degree would get the idea being conveyed.

Generally, day-long conferences are broken down into time sequences for each activity, and participants and speakers have this explicit contract available to them. If one speaker goes beyond his designated time limit and infringes upon the time allowed for other subsequent topics and speakers, he breaks an explicit contract with the audience as well as with those speakers who follow him on the program. Individuals may display hostile behavior toward him and, in a postconference evaluation, communicate their displeasure with his behavior. They may label his behavior arrogant, disrespectful, and selfish. The injustice may *not* be looked upon with such disfavor if sufficient time is available for others to present their material as planned.

All encounters involve a time dimension. Therefore explicit rules relative to total time and the sequencing and synchronization of verbal exchanges among group members should be established prior to initiating group discourse.

Setting or Situation

Socially and culturally defined and accepted rules have been established for various group interactions and social occasions. For example, laughter and joke telling on serious occasions such as during a funeral are considered inappropriate communication behavior. When silence is implied during a church service, and a baby cries and breaks the silence, one may feel some animosity toward the parents of the child. The irritation is often compounded when a nursery service is available to the parents.

Some types of verbal exchange and actions are expected in one situation but would be considered improper in another context. The lawyer, during cross-examination of a witness, and the debater, when trying to make his point, may belittle the opponent into anger and submission. On such occasions this disrespect is acceptable and implied in the rules of the communication game.

Rewards

We engage in communication activity with others for a purpose and expect some personal and/or group gains or rewards from it. Humans are generally too selfish and egocentric not to expect some personal returns from their expenditure of money, time, or effort. The student who chooses to attend an evening guest lecture on campus in lieu of catching up on his studies may feel that the implied contract has been broken if he receives no new information and therefore no benefit or reward from the encounter.

There is a wide range of rewards or benefits individuals may expect from interpersonal communication. They may expect to be entertained, to gain social pleasure, to be stimulated by new knowledge and discovery of new ideas. They may expect to accomplish a goal through group activity which was not possible to experience individually. Any or all of their basic needs of identity, stimulation, and security may be expected to be met to some degree through the relationship and communication with others. The prestige of being asked to meet with a group as their expert consultant may be a reward in itself.

All interpersonal communication involves a *contract* that dictates the expected communication behavior of members of the group. The terms of the contract are operating whether or not all members of the group are aware of them. Whether the contract is explicit or implied, a violation of any of the rules of the encounter can be expected to be reflected in the communication behavior of those experiencing the insult. Factors that enter into the communication contract are expectations or assumptions regarding the purpose and the related content and title of the encounter, the psychological climate and relationship among members, the verbal and the spatial and temporal language, appropriate behavior for the particular setting or situation, and the rewards to be gained.

As a means of summarizing and clarifying some of the aspects of the communication contract, an example of a continuing education program is presented as Figure 6-1. Many *explicit* commitments are readily apparent. A definitive purpose is outlined for participants, and the content, in most cases, is reflected in the title assigned to each scheduled activity for the two day conference. The continuing education units (CEU) the participants will earn for their attendance at the sessions represent the explicit reward. Some implicit rewards or gains might also be expected. For example, the audience would undoubtedly expect to gain new knowledge, and the speakers may expect some personal satisfaction from sharing information as well as a monetary reward that may be explicitly or implicitly arranged prior to the sessions. The title of each activity may or may not dictate the spatial language or relationship expected among members. The time schedule for all activities is clear and definite. Many programmers elect not to expose themselves to such rigid time schedules because of the pressures that result from the need to keep their time commitments.

The reader is encouraged to further explore terms of the contractual agreement represented by the printed program (Figure 6-1). What additional assumptions and expectations would you have as you entered the 2-day conference? What would you expect of others, and what could they logically expect from you regarding communication with one another? Become introspective and reflect on the kinds of behavior you might exhibit if a breach of contract resulted.

If a member of a group not only breaks a term of the agreement but also fails to excuse himself for the infraction, his behavior may well be viewed as a double insult. It is one thing to be forced to wait for one late member to

NURSING LEADERSHIP:
CONTENT, PROCESS and PRACTICE

GENERAL INFORMATION

This program is designed to provide registered nurses with an opportunity to strengthen and up-date knowledge and skills relative to leadership roles. This workshop is Part I of a three part sequence of nursing leadership workshops planned over a three year period; content will focus on leadership needs in work settings, behavioral and situational aspects of nursing leadership and leadership responsibilities relating to nursing issues.

Thursday, June 7, 1973

Morning Session

9:00 a.m. WELCOME_____ R.N., Ph.D.

GOALS OF WORKSHOP
_____R.N., Ph.D.

9:30 a.m. LEADERSHIP NEEDS EXISTING IN NURSE SETTINGS _____R.N., Ed.D.

10:00 Coffee

10:30 THE HUMAN COMMUNICATION GAMBLE_____ R.N., Ph.D.

11:15 COOPERATIVE SQUARES
_____R.N., Ph.D.

12:15 p.m. Lunch

Afternoon Session

1:30 p.m. THE LEADERSHIP PROCESS_____R.N., Ed.D.

2:15 Coffee

2:45 ESTABLISHING THE CLIMATE OF LEADERSHIP___R.N., Ed.D.

3:30 SUMMARY_____R.N., Ph.D.

3:45 ADJOURN

Friday, June 8, 1973

Morning Session

9.00 a.m. SYSTEMS VARIABLES AFFECTING LEADERSHIP____R.N., Ph.D.

9:45 GROUP INTERACTION

10:45 Coffee

11:15 "FEEDBACK" AND DISCUSSION
_____R.N., Ph.D.

12:15 p.m. Lunch

Afternoon Session

1:30 p.m. LEADERSHIP RESPONSIBLITY AND NURSING ISSUES
_____R.N., Ed.D.

3:00 Coffee

3:30 SUMMARY AND EVALUATION___R.N., Ph.D.

3:45 ADJOURN

CREDIT: Continuing Education Programs offered by the College of Nursing will be awarded Continuing Education Units and a permanent record of your participation will be on file. The proposed nation-wide standard of measurement for participation in continuing education programs is THE CONTINUING EDUCATION UNIT (CEU). This program will qualify for 1.0 CEU. The CEU is defined as: TEN CONTACT HOURS OF PARTICIPATION IN AN ORGANIZED CONTINUING EDUCATION EXPERIENCE UNDER RESPONSIBLE SPONSORSHIP, CAPABLE DIRECTION, AND QUALIFIED INSTRUCTION.

Figure 6-1 An explicit communication contract.

arrive and another thing to have that individual fail to either acknowledge or apologize for his failure to meet his obligation. While most of our interpersonal communication takes place as an informal social encounter, when more formal groups meet it is well for the members to mutually formulate and accept the rules of communication behavior prior to further interaction if effective communication is desired.

SUGGESTED BIBLIOGRAPHY

Flesch, Rudolf: *The Art of Readable Writing,* Collier-Macmillan, London, 1949.
Howe, Reuel L.: *The Miracle of Dialogue,* The Seabury Press, New York, 1963.
Wiemann, John M. and Mark L. Knapp.: "Turn-taking in Conversations," *Journal of Communication*, **25**(2):75–92, Spring 1975.

Chapter 7

Dysfunctional
Communication:
Barriers and Bridges

I must do these things in order to communication: Become aware of you (discover you). Make you aware of me (uncover myself). Be ready to change during our conversation, and be willing to reveal my changes to you.

Hugh Prather

Dysfunctional communication is an endemic social disease in American society. At times it reaches epidemic proportions, when individuals and groups flaunt their distaste for certain rules and regulations by participating in riots and sit-ins. The term *dysfunctional* will be used in the context of this discussion to mean failure either to get a response to a message or to get the response the sender expected. The messages may be regarded as confusing, conflicting, or obscure.

We spend much of our lives polluting messages. Generally this is done out of ignorance rather than malice, and often it is done out of awareness. However, the intent generally has little bearing on the consequences of the disturbed communication that results. The barriers to communication are ultimately the participants themselves, for communication is a people process. We might paraphrase the statement "Many thought it was the apple on the tree that caused all of the trouble when it really was the pair on the ground" to read "Many thought it was the word used in the sentence that caused the communication problem rather than the human responses to it." It is the person, not the word, who bears the message meaning, just as it is the driver, not the red light, who stops the car!

It is obvious that the solution cannot be one of getting rid of people or even of making any major and lasting changes in the way in which they behave. Our focus must be directed toward the means of eliminating the barriers permanently where that might be possible and bridging some of the problems. Because of the complexities and the transactional nature of the human communication process, no single barrier operates in isolation, nor are single solutions or bridges readily effective. The difficulty inherent in bridging the communication barriers becomes apparent when we realize that the solution resides, to a major extent, in those who created the problem.

BARRIERS

Communication barriers in general stem from the fact that we do not fully understand and/or appreciate the complex human communication process and are not in tune with ourselves or with those with whom we attempt to communicate. While our language is inadequate at best, we continually nourish the semantic bacteria, both the verbal and the nonverbal bugs, that invade and infect our human communication system.

Communication is essential to life, yet it is discouraging and frustrating to find repeated barriers that alienate individuals from one another. We also experience intrapersonal communication barriers that may affect our psychological and social functioning. There are no *absolute* barriers. An identified barrier in one situation may be present but cause no problem to communication in another situation. However, there are a number of *potential* barriers that more frequently than others produce dysfunctional communication. Some of these will be discussed here. The reader is asked to insert a mental subscript "(potential)" each time the word "barrier" is used.

Most of the barriers are psychological rather than physiological. *Physical* barriers are those primarily related to sensory dysfunction. The blind and/or deaf individual has lost the sensory acuity needed to begin the processing of messages. Nothing can be perceived until it is sensed, as evident from the intrapersonal communication model and as discussed previously. Physiological perceptual disorders may also cause dysfunctional communication. Anyone who has ever tried to engage in verbal discourse with an individual who has had his larynx removed knows of some of the barriers that exist. Not only may the message be difficult to understand because of distorted sound, but emotional barriers may also be present because of the stress and frustration experienced by either or both parties. Physiological or mechanical anomalies of the mouth, nose, or any other speech organs might be expected to produce dysfunctional communication as well.

Noise is any extraneous, spurious, undesirable, or unintended stimulus. It may result from channel overload and may distort the perception and processing of messages. Noise has message quality but may produce stress and disturbance to our nervous system and become a barrier to intrapersonal and interpersonal communication. There is no pure or absolute noise. In fact, one man's noise may be another man's message. For example, to the viewer, the *snow* or distorted television picture, may be noise, but to the television repairman it is an important message that assists him in detecting the trouble.

There may be internal or external noise. *Internal noise* may come from the individual's programmed attitudes, values, interests, and needs system. Many rigid individuals get caught in their own cocoon, and the noise caused by their inner control system obscures or confuses external messages. The internal filter system may be so strong as to appear as noise along with all external messages. There may be the physiological noise of fatigue, illness, stress, or pain. Noise may result from differences, associated with space and time factors, between individuals from different cultures.

External noise may result from messages being sent on several channels simultaneously. For example, a mother may be talking with a neighbor while her child is pulling at her apron to get her attention. Irritating repetition, incessant chatter, and the static from a radio are further examples of noise barriers. Because we can attend to only one message at a time, all other potential messages have the possibility of being barriers to communication.

Redundancy consists of sending more than a single cue to express an idea. The same thought may be conveyed with a variety of words and/or on various channels. The most elementary form of redundancy is mere repetition. The degree and type of redundancy determine whether it will be perceived as noise and thus be a barrier to the intended message. When an individual views the repetition as unnecessary, excessive, and irritating, it may be noise. Some redundancy is essential in all communication, but "too much," which is in part an individual matter, may serve as a barrier. Our English language itself is said to be 50 percent redundant. In face-to-face encounters, nonverbal messages accompany verbal messages and there may be some redundancy. Some of the barriers to family communication are attributable to "preaching" and "nagging" that are so redundant as to be noise.

When two messages are expressed and one of them denies the other, the result is labeled a *double bind*. It is a potential communication barrier. At some time or another, we have all had the experience of being confused in our interpretation of messages that seem to be conflicting, in which symbols are at variance with one another. Incongruent messages create double binds. We might paraphrase a Lucy-to-Charlie-Brown statement as "You're a good concept, double bind, if only you weren't so wishy-washy."

The most frequent dichotomies occur between verbal and nonverbal messages or statements that themselves hold contradictions. For example, one might verbalize his love for someone but display dislike and disgust through his posture and facial expressions. Or a sign may read "We welcome your suggestions; place them here," and the "here" is over the wastepaper basket. Then there are the individuals who proclaim their democratic approach to problem solving and ask for suggestions, when they have already initiated a plan of action. "Here I am again for the first time" is an example of a contradiction within a verbal statement. Due to some conventional meaning we place on words, "dry lakes" and "fish farms" may irritate our nervous system and be labeled double binds.

Man is a complex organism, and people frequently exhibit behaviors that are contradictory or at least appear so to others. Yet because we are rational beings, one's behavior may make sense to oneself even though it does not seem congruent to others. Double binds can occur in any types of relationship and are particularly common in family communication. As they relate to dysfunctional communication, the question is whether the double binds are *patterns* of communication interaction or just periodic and isolated occurrences. In a study of schizophrenic children, it was found that the mothers of those children tended to be ambiguous and evasive in their communication behavior. Their children had difficulty discriminating and determining the true message. Emotional disturbance resulted from the double binds. It was theorized that schizophrenic individuals find the world so confusing that they withdraw into their own world.[1]

All double binds are not pathogenic. Double binds are used in our humor and in the creative process. Some paradoxes must be tolerated. Husbands and wives often create double-bind situations but over the years learn to cope with them. One may accommodate by withdrawing, by "hearing" only part of the message, by disqualifying the statement as symptomatic behavior, or by giving a dual message in reply as a humorous remark. The feminist movement and the study of equal rights for women

---

[1]David H. Olson, "Empirically Unbinding the Double Bind: Review of Research and Conceptual Reformulations," *Family Process*, 11(1):69–94, March 1972.

have unveiled many double binds in our communication system, between what is written or declared and what is observed in practice.

Individuals sending messages may not be aware of the contradictions that others read from their messages. This is particularly true of people communicating cross-culturally. For example, there was a foreign woman who was asked what she thought of Americans. Her reply was: "They are funny people. They make a drink and put whiskey in to warm them up and ice to cool them down; lemon to make it sour and soda to make it sweet; then lift the glass in the air, say 'Here's to you,' and drink it themselves— funny people!"

Our verbal language is loaded with potential barriers, many of which have been brought on by an Aristotelian orientation. This orientation has resulted in misevaluations because of the assumed two-valued (either/or) and static system. Careless *generalizations* and groupings have led to distorted communication. For example, the Gray Panthers, an organization of senior citizens, has tried to monitor the way the elderly have been portrayed on television: as people tied to rocking chairs. "The establishment" and "hippies" are but some of the many stereotyped labels assigned to individuals and groups. In the discussion of general semantics, the Aristotelian philosophy will be discussed in more detail as it relates to human communication.

Habit is a strong potential communication barrier. We do so many things habitually that when someone calls our behavior to our attention, we feel awkward in trying to change. For example, it has been suggested that when you find that your golf partner is consistently out-distancing you with his drive and your chances of winning are slim, you should just bring his swing into his conscious state of awareness by saying, "Gee, John, I'm surprised you hit the ball so well; you don't seem to be bringing your club head back far enough." Then watch his next swing. As Prather observed, "Tonight at dinner I tried picking up my glass with my left hand instead of my right and I didn't feel quite so self-assured."[2] Prather also said: "In order to break with a habit I will first have to become aware of how I usually act. I will have to see how I do it before I can undo it. At the time, I am not aware of how I shut down my attention or hold back my warmth."[3] His statements clearly point out some of the many ways in which habit can get in the way of effective communication. We may be reluctant to admit that we have rigid and established patterns in our behavior which foster dysfunctional communication.

Dogmatism, or closed-mindedness, is a serious potential barrier because of the constricting limits placed on data inputs. The rigid controls reduce one's ability to change and grow. The dogmatic individual is

[2]Prather, *I Touch the Earth, the Earth Touches Me*.
[3]Prather, *I Touch the Earth, the Earth Touches Me*.

reluctant to take in any data contradictory to his programmed inner system. He is generally difficult to persuade, shows limited creative ability, and is unwilling to accept or even consider alternative interpretations. He is an excellent candidate for what Toffler has labeled *future shock*.[4] Messages that touch on the individual's central beliefs are particularly difficult for him to consider.

The dogmatic individual is generally impulsive, defensive, and stereotyped in his thinking and interpersonal communication behavior. He generally lacks flexibility and is conservative in his views. The closed-minded individual's response to messages usually is based more on his perception of the message *source* than on the message content. He tends to seek out individuals in a group who conform to his own belief system and sees wide disparity between his belief system and the views of those who disagree with him. He leads a life of self-justification. Not only is his behavior self-destructive, but also his insensitivity and intolerance of others serve as a barrier to encounters in the groups of which he is a member.

An unfortunate aspect of being in a group in which there are closed-minded individuals who make very rigid dogmatic remarks is the tendency for other members to reciprocate with dogmatic responses. The negative behavior of others triggers similar behavior in us. As Harris explained it, we *react rather than act*; we lose control and let others push our button.[5] As we react, we become increasingly vulnerable to manipulation by others. If and when we become aware that other group members are controlling our behavior, we may be inclined to direct hostile behavior toward them. It is quite evident that the interpersonal communication in such a group would be highly dysfunctional.

The *assumptions* made relating to communication are legion. It is difficult to eliminate our assumptive world because we are often unaware of how our behavior is based on false, untested, unquestioned, and consequently unresolved assumptions. Many of our assumptive errors are a reflection of lack of understanding of the communication process, the means by which messages are sensed, perceived, and transformed into symbolic meaning. A few of the common assumptions upon which communication behavior is based are that we live in a static rather than a dynamic state, that words are the thing rather than a representation of it, that meaning is in words rather than in people, and that individuals have like perceptions. We assume that added talk will automatically result in greater probability of effective communication.

The assumptions we bring to a situation become critical factors affecting communication. We fare no better than the ants who make false

[4]Toffler, *Future Shock*.
[5]Sydney J. Harris, *Last Things First*, Houghton Mifflin Co., Boston, 1957, pp. 2–3.

assumptions about "dead" ants: It seems that when an ant dies, a substance or odor is released, other ants get the message that the ant has died, and they carry it away. A research study was done whereby this substance was placed on *live* ants. Before long, without checking out their assumptions, the other ants dragged these live ants away because they were *assumed* to be dead. The moral of the story might be that people, like ants, get into trouble by making assumptions that they then act upon without testing them. Wendell Johnson pointed out a similar problem of mice. He said that mousetraps were successful because cheese was cheese—always food and never bait.[6]

We make assumptions as we *fill voids*. There was the story of two men who were driving along a country road when they came upon a herd of sheep. One of the men remarked "Gee, that's a lovely herd of sheared sheep," to which the other man replied, "Well, they are sheared on *this* side." Too often we see a part of something and assume that it is representative of the whole. Many misevaluations are made because of unquestioned assumptions and a tendency to fill in the voids of missing data. We hear part of a conversation and fill in the rest. Someone starts a sentence, and we finish it for him as we expect *he* would finish it. Sometimes we both ask *and* answer the question for the other person. We may not hear the response because of what we expected the person to say. All of this may happen without our being consciously aware of it, at least until someone responds in a different way than we had expected. Rumors and grapevines develop from our practice of filling in the missing data.

Three men were looking at an elephant, obviously from their own unique frame of reference. The dentist said, "Gee, what a lovely tusk of ivory!" The hunter's remark was, "What a nice trophy head for my game room!" The businessman remarked, "It reminds me of my mother-in-law, ——!" How many of you quickly filled the void with assumptions relative to the weight of the mother-in-law? His comment actually was, "She's a Republican." How quickly our minds work to complete a thought, to fill the voids as we expect them to be filled—and how often we are wrong! All too frequently we become mesmerized with words and fail to respond to our senses. How often individuals will eat buffalo meat or horsemeat with delight until someone labels it "buffalo meat" or "horsemeat!"

We pollute and distort messages when using technical language or *jargon* that is not known by all. Technical or secret language adopted for use by a specific discipline, for example, can divide people and create psychological distance. Jargon might be viewed as a part of the *territorial defense* which designates membership in a particular subculture. The intent of communication is to breed understanding, yet the indiscriminate use of jargon may do just the opposite. "Cerebral cortical endowment not

[6]Johnson, *People in Quandaries*.

exactly excessive'' is a reflection of medical jargon that implies a ''dumb'' individual in lay terms. Anyone who has changed from one field of study to a very divergent one realizes that it may take months just to become familiar with the unique language of the new discipline. As well as verbal jargon, there is nonverbal jargon that is equally difficult to understand.

Inherent in *written messages* is an uncertainty not present in face-to-face communication. Missing is the important nonverbal aspect that generally accompanies verbal messages. The absence of *immediate* feedback to correct and clarify messages also makes written messages more prone to misevaluation. Individuals actually alienate themselves from others through the physical and psychological distance of written messages. ''A printed speech is like a dried flower: the substance, indeed, is there, but the color is faded and the perfume gone'' (Paul Lorain). The written message is sterile when compared with the intimacy of face-to-face encounters.

From the previous discussion of the communication-trust-risk paradigm, it should be evident that *distrust* between individuals, or even a lack of trust or confidence in self, may result in dysfunctional communication. When an individual or group feels powerless to affect its own destiny and is suspicious and distrustful of others, the rumor and grapevine mills work overtime. It has been said that ''Some grapevines are so bad that they have root rot!'' In a large organization in which there is only one-way communication and that is done primarily through written directives, the only defense individual employees may have is to open their own channels of communication and fill the voids by making assumptions to accommodate for the missing data. Withholding and distorting of information are symptomatic of distrust within a group.

Other barriers to communication result from our being ill-equipped to deal with or be aware of the importance played by our *nonverbal language*. Our mobile and global society creates regional and cultural barriers that often leave us insensitive to others and having communication problems.

Individuals may withdraw from encounters with others from the fear of both being understood and being *misunderstood*. The eight terms of the interpersonal communication contract also produce dysfunctional communication if any one is not met.

The barriers to communication are innumerable. Those just given are but a few of the most common ones we find operating as we relate to ourselves and others. Many barriers are out of awareness, necessitating our first bringing them to the conscious level before remedies can be applied.

BRIDGES

If better communication is our goal, we must do something about the way we relate to ourselves and others. For example, the researcher and the practitioner as the consumer of research must establish an effective two-way flow of information or neither one will successfully fulfill his commitment to himself and society. While we may all accept the need to live happily and productively with others, many of us are not willing to expend the effort to reach that goal. The only alternative may be to heed former President Harry S. Truman's advice, "If you want a friend in this world, get a dog."

There are the perennial pessimists who say that with such a galaxy of potential barriers, there is little chance of our ever reaching a state of effective communication. Some individuals may elect to withdraw from any attempts to improve and may continue with their haphazard hit-and-miss approach. In facing the problems, we must direct our attention to *prevention*, as we must do in health care. Treatment of the ills of communication, as with the physical and emotional ills of life, is too costly in time, money, and effort. To remedy the infirmities that have resulted from such barriers as lack of trust or false assumptions is an expensive and difficult task.

Most of the barriers are created by people. They may not be aware of or understand the communication process. They may fail in getting in touch with self or developing sensitivity to those with whom they attempt to communicate. Some of the best bridges to effective communication revolve around feelings of basic human dignity and respect for others.

Businesses and other organizations in increasing numbers are employing human communication methodologists and consultants to identify and deal with potential communication problems within the organization. A *communication consultant* plays the role of "social engineer," applying basic knowledge to improving everyday human communication behavior. The consultant may help resolve group conflict, facilitate ideation and social change, encourage creativity, and foster more effective and efficient problem solving. He may assist personnel at all levels of the organization to become more aware of the potential barriers that impede their progress toward desired goals.

Identifying the barriers may be a first step, but it is not enough. The barriers must be eliminated, reduced, or replaced. While stereotypes, biases, and prejudices may not be successfully outlawed, other potential barriers can be eliminated through honest dialogue. The communication of respect, acceptance, and understanding can replace the negative effects of suspicion, biases, and stereotypes. Many of the bridges are directed toward fostering interpersonal accord.

There are methodologies and training sessions geared toward increasing one's *self-awareness*. EST, assertiveness training, biofeedback, and human relations laboratories are some examples. Everyone must be encouraged to become more *introspective*; to learn of his own personal biography, values, stereotypes, needs, and ways his behavior affects and is affected by others. If we could only become aware, through the reflection in the mirror, of the barriers we set up, we might be one step closer to ridding our system of dysfunctional communication. However, as Huxley said, "Ye shall know the truth and the truth shall make ye mad." It is difficult to look at the truth about ourself. "Nature didn't make us perfect so she did the next best thing—she made us blind to our own faults."*

Self-discovery is the only learning that really influences behavior. Know thyself—foster psychological introspection. Books are filled with communication games to help individuals get in touch with self. Exploring one's response to such simple questions as "Who *am* I?" or "If you had a 25-hour today, how would you spend it?" can do much to get at the basis upon which we communicate.

In the past, the internal milieu, while admittedly significant, was considered to be difficult if not impossible to control. The focus therefore centered on efforts to improve the external communication environment. The popular biofeedback, a means of training individuals to control their internal behavior is now available.

Building *self-confidence* is a bridge to more effective intrapersonal and interpersonal communication. One could "psych oneself up" by following the notion that individuals use only 15 percent of their potential. If each of us could bring himself to activate the 85 percent of the ability he has in reserve, at least his self-confidence might be improved.

It is a fact that while we may be liked by some people, we will not be liked by others. So why not be ourselves and stop trying so hard to impress others by putting on a facade? Putting away phoniness and being *genuine* is a solid bridge to interpersonal communication. Communication with others can improve if we make our inner and outer feelings and expressions congruent. An example of this was of a young woman who was attending a large group session at an American Nurses' Association convention. During the open discussion she stood up, and before she began to make her point she revealed her true inner feelings. She said that she was frightened and felt quite humble about making her thoughts known before such a large group of "experts" and well-known individuals. She made no attempt to mask her uncomfortable feeling, and by the time she got to express her views she had gained the compassion and empathic understanding of the group. She also tended to become more relaxed after revealing herself to the group. We seldom view the expression of feelings as a means of strengthening a relationship, yet that is what happened here. To hold back feelings of fear or anger is to accept the choice of destroying self rather than the relationship.

Another bridge we must try to build is *sensitivity to others*. It requires

*Quotations not attributed to a specific source were gathered by the author from various places.

empathic understanding. There are limits as to how closely we can "feel with others," but the more congruent our perceptions, the greater the chances for effective interpersonal communication. Women have been found to be more sensitive and interpersonally aware than men, but empathic ability is a bridge worthy of being built by all. Too often we criticize another individual and make verbal attacks upon him because we fail to understand his internal environment. By establishing *dialogue* we can bridge the physical and psychological distance between people. One of President Carter's campaign promises was kept on Inauguration Day in January 1977, when he got out of his limousine and he and his wife and family walked the distance from the capitol to the viewing stand to symbolically and literally establish closeness with the American people. His physical exposure on that historic walk also symbolized his *trust* in the people.

Our *verbal language* warrants our attention and respect, for it is involved in many of the potential barriers to communication. Words must be treated for what they are: mere arbitrarily derived symbols, or representations, of people and objects. Some semantic barriers can be eliminated if we minimize the use of words that tend to convey extremes in meaning. There is a common saying, " 'Never' and 'always' are two words one should *always* remember *never* to use" and a similar "rule," "Always avoid 'always' and never say 'never.' " Sometimes simple substitutions of words can make the difference between attaining effective communication or not attaining it. For example, the word "many" might be preferable to "all," "usually" to "always," "seldom" to "never," "similar" to "the same," and "among other things" to "only." A semantic awareness to words that have a tendency to cause negative reactions in others must be developed.

When we mean "I want you to," little is gained by cloaking our meaning in the words "You ought to." Frequently better results are obtained if we inform ("I am not finished") rather than order ("Stop interrupting me"). It was Oliver Wendell Holmes who was concerned about people trying to impress others by using big words. He said, "Some men ligate arteries; others tie them and it stops bleeding just as well." Additional suggestions for bridging potential semantic barriers will be presented later in this chapter, in the discussion of general semantics.

Feedback is a control or regulatory mechanism whereby the source can obtain information regarding the effect his message is having on the receiver. It makes communication a circular rather than a simple linear process. If the source of the original message is aware of the feedback to his message, he may elect to correct or modify subsequent messages in an effort to increase his chances of getting the intended message across. There is greater uncertainty when there is no feedback or when individuals are insensitive and/or unresponsive to it. Feedback is immediate and is generally more useful as a bridge to communication when it comes from a face-to-face encounter instead of from a printed memo or written discourse. The reaction of the receiver actually becomes a message going back to the original source telling him where he stands in terms of effective communication. When a double bind becomes a barrier to communication, immediate feedback may provide the bridge by means of which to ask for a message clarification and/or alert the sender of the double message he is sending. To seek clarification of the double bind, one must be willing to risk actually losing the relationship. The more dependent the individuals are in the relationship in which the double-bind message occurs, the greater is the resistance to asking for clarification of the message. *Role playing* is a programmed form of feedback designed to help individuals see and feel how their communication behavior affects others. Tape recorders and video tapes provide recorded feedback for more complete analysis.

Redundancy has already been presented as a potential barrier to effective communication. It may also serve as a means of reducing the ambiguity and uncertainty of messages. Mere repetition may more likely be a barrier, while redundancy experienced on various channels may serve to enhance communication. Whether redundancy will be a barrier or a bridge to communication depends upon the individual's tolerance of and need for it. Limited redundancy generally will reduce potential transmission errors. Nonverbal messages accompanying verbal utterances may help clarify and reinforce messages. Generally the written word requires less redundancy than the spoken word because there is less noise involved.

Extra or redundant cues are provided so that the message will have a better chance to penetrate, despite the noise, and provide varied stimuli to the sensory receptors. When the source is sending messages to a heterogeneous audience, more redundancy may be needed to reach the audience's wide range of differences in comprehension. In such cases one always runs the risk of having the redundancy become *noise* to those who did not need it for comprehension of the message.

Redundancy is a bridge to help ensure against message error. Basically we are trying to increase our odds in the communication gamble by providing additional stimuli. Doing this is analogous to throwing out many balls in attempting to increase our chances of hitting the target.

"True eloquence consists in saying all that is necessary, and nothing but what is necessary" (La Rochefoucauld). That would be a good rule to follow if only we knew exactly how much was *necessary* for each individual! The Viking Space Program was patterned with a great deal of redundancy to accommodate for the possibility of system malfunctioning. So it is with the redundancy in our communication system. Associations in our cognitive process are strengthened by repetition and redundancy.

Listening is a very active part of interpersonal communication and can be a bridge to effective functioning. "Know how to listen and you will profit even from those who talk badly," advised Plutarch. Listening is much more than audition. It is channeling one's attention and staying quiet inside. It requires the reduction or elimination of internal and external noise or distractions. Nonverbal messages as well as the verbal ones must be attended to. We must "listen" to words, sequence of phrases, silences, posture, tone of voice, eye movement, and a plethora of other verbal and nonverbal cues. Prather said: "I believe that at least one of the reasons why prayer, relaxation drills, yoga, self-hypnotism, tai chi, breathing concentration and Gestalt awareness exercises bring peace and dissolve problems is that they force an end to the merry-go-round of thinking. Either during or after these meditations we do something rare: we stop and listen."[7]

Efforts must be made to *open the minds of dogmatic individuals* in a group who are rigid in their belief that their knowledge is complete and infallible and therefore they do not have to be open to new inputs. In a *climate of trust*, in which members can openly admit their faults and errors and make fun of themselves, individuals can feel freer to admit that they need new inputs. They must look at the feasibility of *always* being right versus being human, where erring is an inherent trait. Group efforts must be directed toward helping closed-minded individuals accept the realities of a dynamic state rather than the static base from which they tend to operate. Some principles of general semantics relating to this area will be discussed in more detail later.

Intensive interactions with others may help reduce the limited view of dogmatic individuals. Some individuals are more tactful and skilled than others in helping others adopt new norms and response patterns. Promoting a healthy relationship is important: "It is hard for a fellow to keep a chip on his shoulder if you allow him to take a bow." Facts may help dislodge a person's misevaluations, unless of course he is too rigid to even look at his misguided way of viewing the world.

Transaction Analysis was designed as a contractual form of therapy,[8] and some of its concepts may serve as a bridge to effective communication. The contract represents an individual's commitment to himself and other group members that he will make some specific changes in his communication patterns. The expected behavior fits the rules of the contract, and attention is drawn to that behavior during the encounters.

In some group situations, communication may be improved if individuals can be *made aware of* how their mood and behavior affects others in the group. The *reciprocal effect* their behavior has on others triggers

[7]Prather, *I Touch the Earth, the Earth Touches Me*.

[8]Muriel James and Dorothy Jongeward, *Born to Win: Transactional Analysis with Gestalt Experiments,* Addison-Wesley Publishing Co., Reading, Mass., 1971.

reactions in them. In the same way, individuals can very easily make *their* problems become the problems of the group. Individuals must be confronted with their behavior and its effect on group goals. Children are especially gifted at conveying ownership of their problems to their parents, who unwittingly accept them.

The bridges proposed to span some of the identified potential barriers are presented as suggestions and are not to be construed as all-inclusive. There is no instant cures or patent medicines to alleviate communication barriers. Some bridges provided through the methodology of general semantics are presented as a final suggested approach for individuals to follow.

GENERAL SEMANTICS AS A DESCRIPTIVE AND PRESCRIPTIVE DISCIPLINE

General semantics provides one way of studying the etiology of communication disorders. It focuses on the relationship between man's use of language and the way he thinks and behaves. General semantics is a descriptive and prescriptive discipline that has much to offer in the way of improving our intrapersonal and interpersonal communication. The methodology proposed can help eliminate barriers and also provide preventive means for improving our functioning. It involves training in social skills.

General semantics is concerned with the sanity of the race. It involves the study of the environment within people. While there are no gimmicks involved, it provides unlimited help in personal and social adjustment. It is a rational and practical methodology to be used by the individual himself to gain control over his external and internal environments. It explains and trains us in how to better use our nervous system. There is an old adage that says, "God may forgive you your sins, but your nervous system won't."

Alfred Korzybski is regarded as the "father" of general semantics. The original source book of general semantics was his classic, *Science and Sanity*, which was first published in 1933.[9] His first work, *Manhood of Humanity*, was published in 1922.[10] It was Korzybski's belief that the structure of language affects the functioning of our nervous system, that words elicit internal responses that he labeled *semantic reactions*. He disagreed with the Laws of Aristotle and blamed some maladjustment of individuals on Aristotelian orientation and training.

General semantics is primarily geared toward releasing individuals from their traditional Aristotelian training. In fact, the symbol for general

---

[9]Korzybski, *Science and Sanity*.

[10]Alfred Korzybski, *Manhood of Humanity*, 2d ed., The International Non-Aristotelian Library Publishing Co., Lakeville, Conn., 1950.

semantics is Ā, which is symbolic of a non-Aristotelian approach to the evaluation and structuring of our language. General semantics is prescribed as a means of analyzing, understanding, and improving human communication in any field of human endeavor. Its principles have been applied to medicine, law, education, business, and virtually every facet of everyday life. It is indispensable for medicine in general and psychiatry and mental health in particular. It is presented as a discipline capable of developing more mature human behavior and eliminating some of the semantic bacteria from our system.

Only a brief presentation of the concepts, theories, and methodology of general semantics can be presented here. The reader is encouraged to delve more deeply into study of this field. It is an exciting, viable, and pragmatic approach to learning about our reaction to language and the means whereby we can reduce some of the misevaluations that get in the way of effective communication with ourselves and others.

Abstracting is a normal part of the communication process, yet most of the time we abstract without being aware of it. It is a chain of associations we make as a response to a stimulus from the environment. As we move upward on the chain or *abstracting ladder*, we get further away from the nonverbal, extensional, factual, and feeling levels and more onto the verbal, intensional, and inferential levels (Figure 7-1). On the nonverbal level we refer to a *specific* object without using verbal labels, but as we proceed into the verbal levels we move increasingly farther from facts and specifics to inferences and generalities. We make inferences about inferences and selectively, and generally unconsciously, omit many of the unique characteristics of the object at the higher orders of abstraction. At high verbal levels we group and categorize objects, people, and events for convenience. While we consider the similarities among them in the process of grouping, we commit gross misevaluations because we tend to avoid significant differences.

The whole system of general semantics is based on the theory that by *becoming conscious* of abstracting, we can select more mature behavior, reduce our chances of misevaluation, and correct many of our linguistic barriers to communication. Not only is it imperative that we be aware of the level at which *we* are abstracting at a particular time, but in our encounters with others we must also be aware of *their* order of abstraction. Controversy is confusion over levels of abstraction.

If two individuals are *shown* a thin, 6-inch-long plastic object with a metal clip, they are receiving a nonverbal stimulus and there is a good possibility that it would elicit congruent meaning between them. However, we are verbal animals, and we quickly assign labels to objects as we move onto the *intensional* verbal levels where congruent meaning becomes less of a possibility than at the nonverbal level. Now each individual is asked to

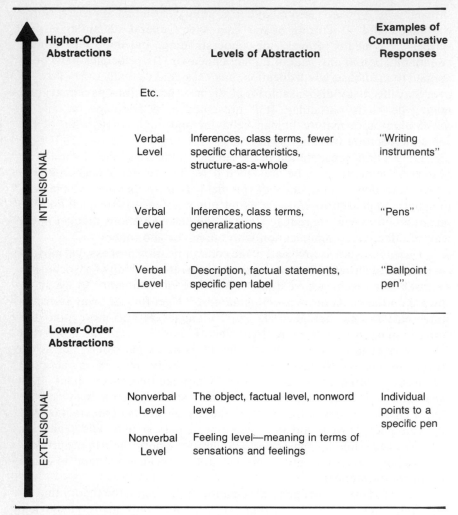

	Higher-Order Abstractions	Levels of Abstraction	Examples of Communicative Responses
	Etc.		
INTENSIONAL	Verbal Level	Inferences, class terms, fewer specific characteristics, structure-as-a-whole	"Writing instruments"
	Verbal Level	Inferences, class terms, generalizations	"Pens"
	Verbal Level	Description, factual statements, specific pen label	"Ballpoint pen"
	Lower-Order Abstractions		
EXTENSIONAL	Nonverbal Level	The object, factual level, nonword level	Individual points to a specific pen
	Nonverbal Level	Feeling level—meaning in terms of sensations and feelings	

Figure 7-1   The abstracting process.

independently and quickly write down in ascending order the four to five words that come to mind when they look at the object. A comparison of the words each individual wrote down as his association process at each level can help point out how uniquely each individual abstracts and how much abstraction can be a barrier to communication. For example, referring to Figure 7-1, if one of the individuals was at the first verbal level with the words "ballpoint pen" while the second individual was at a higher level at which he categorized the object under the label "writing instruments," one might expect confusion and/or conflict as they attempted to communicate with one another. The second individual might hand the other one a pencil (writing instrument) when a ballpoint pen was expected. This example might help explain why an individual's communication behavior appears totally rational to the person himself but may make little sense to another individual. The significance of the abstracting process to interpersonal communication might be intensified and reinforced in readers if they would engage in a similar experiment with another individual. The variation in abstracting becomes more evident as increasing numbers of individuals compare their patterns of association to a given stimulus.

Ideally we function on all levels of abstraction but must return to the *extensional* nonverbal level from time to time to correct misevaluations made at the higher verbal levels. General semantics proposes ways by which we can delay the labeling and try to stay quiet inside, to stay longer at the extensional level, where there is less chance for misevaluation. It is not easy to look at an object in a room and not attach a label to it, but we can work at it. We can attend to the labels we make, be conscious of our abstracting, and identify where we are on the abstraction ladder.

The methodology of general semantics includes *five delayed, or extensional, devices* that might be viewed as bridges to overcome some of our communication barriers. Each of these will be discussed briefly together with a number of other suggestions offered by general semantics. We get *intensional* as we get caught up in word symbols. There are many defects in the structure of language that we use, and they must not only be brought to our awareness but also changed or eliminated where appropriate. Again, many of our problems have been the result of Aristotelian training, and the antithetical general semantics approach may resolve them.

The five extensional devices proposed are: (1) quotation marks to convey awareness that our abstracting process is unique, (2) dating to acknowledge that the world is dynamic, (3) indexing to reflect acceptance of individual uniqueness, (4) "etc." to acknowledge the fact that we "can never say all about anything," and (5) a hyphen to prevent semantic separation of elements that should be joined.

The implied or explicit use of *quotation marks* or "to-me-ness" statements reflects the ownership of our abstraction and of our statements. EXAMPLE: "*It seems to me* that it would be best to postpone the meeting" is a statement of ownership and is less dogmatic than "Postpone the meeting." Some individuals have used the nonverbal finger gestures symbolic of quotation marks to claim ownership of a verbal statement. Because of the dysfunctional communication that results from dogmatic statements, this extensional device is a worthy suggestion.

Our verbal language must reflect the fact that we live in a dynamic world, where everything and everyone is constantly changing. By *dating* or putting a referent point of time on the statements we make, we open ourselves and others to that change. At the present time something may appear possible, but it may not tomorrow nor did it yesterday. EXAMPLE: "George is ugly." When? "*Today* George is ugly" is a remark that appropriately allows the speaker to be open to perceive a change that may occur at another time and also conveys more of a possibility for that individual to feel the freedom to change. In this particular case, plastic surgery, dental care, new clothes, and cosmetics could do wonders! Our language must reflect that fact. Dating our statements helps us to keep from being locked in with our stereotypes and possibly our need for maintaining self-consistency to such a rigid degree.

Few people will argue with the concept of individuality, yet we fail to reflect it in our verbal and nonverbal language. To remedy the categorical mania that is part of the Aristotelian orientation, we must *index*, or be specific as to, which unique lawyer, doctor, police officer, or schoolteacher we are referring. By giving the same attention to individuals' *differences* as we do to their similarities, their uniqueness will become more apparent. Classifications are high orders of abstraction, and, as such, are unavoidably static as well. No two things or people are ever alike, and therefore things and people should defy being categorized as groups. The ill effects of stereotyping can be eliminated if the uniqueness of individuals is considered. EXAMPLE: "Policemen are cruel" should be replaced by a statement that identifies, by name, unique individual(s) who are cruel. "*Bert Larson* the policeman is cruel." (The statement requires further changes to establish reference to time.)

A basic premise of general semantics is that we "can never say all about anything," for there is always more to be said. The way to reflect this "non-allness" is the use of etc. In fact, the official organ of the International Society for General Semantics is entitled *ETC: A Review of General Semantics*. There are an infinite number of qualities about people and objects, about ways of viewing, and about alternatives to a problem, yet Aristotle presented an either/or polarity to our thought and language processes. *Allness statements*, such as "This is the *only* way it can be done" or "Either we go to the ballgame or we stay home," which relates to the Law of the Excluded Middle, follow Aristotelian concepts and result in communication problems. EXAMPLE: "*One point to make* is that we will need more money" is a verbal expression of the fact that there are other points to be made.

The fifth extensional device is the use of the *hyphen* to keep together concepts, events, or elements that belong together by semantically joining them. EXAMPLE: "Spatial-temporal" rather than "space and time" and "psychosomatic" rather than "mind and body" show the intimate relationship of the elements to one another.

A few additional suggestions general semantics offers as possible bridges to the many barriers we have are presented here. Most of our knowledge comes from *inference*, yet we tend to respond to it as though it were fact. Inference is anything we do not experience directly. That makes our history books loaded with inferential information. It also explains why we get so many different descriptions of the same historic events. The major point to be made is that we *separate inference from fact* and not deal with it as fact.

Is can be a dangerous word. In a certain context it implies a static rather than a dynamic state; it may make a remark an allness statement; and it may reflect a generalization. Using the extensional devices of dating, etc., and indexing, respectively, we can correct the statements to reflect a more accurate world. The semantic reactions of our nervous system to the word "is" are the bases of many of our group dynamics problems.

Definitions provide meager clues as to how an individual will attach meaning to a word. Definitions are mere words about words or symbols of symbols. The meaning resides in people and not in the word. We are easily misled if we place much credence in dictionary definitions, which are merely the history of how a word has been used most frequently in some context at different times. Each word must, of necessity, serve to elicit a vast number of meanings. The number of word symbols man has arbitrarily created is limited. It is not a question of what *it* (word) means but of what *you* mean.

Descriptions and *analogies* have been suggested as a way to convey verbal messages that will have a greater chance of being perceived as intended than dictionary definitions do. *Operational definitions** have also been found to be more useful. Analogies and descriptions increase the chances of attaining isomorphism in meaning because the attempt is made to use something familiar to clarify the unfamiliar. For example, "peace" is a frog resting on a water lily, or a "fortune cookie" is a pizza with cramps.

All of the barriers that have been identified and the bridges suggested to transport us toward effective intrapersonal and interpersonal communication can accomplish little unless they are applied in real life. That becomes my challenge to the reader! An exciting aspect of the study of human communication, as perceived by this author, is that this very minute, tomorrow, and all of the days that follow, each of us can test out these hypotheses in our own human research laboratory. We can try out new ways of relating to others and observe the effect on us and our relationship with them. We can reflect on the semantic reactions from our nervous system and learn more about our thought, behavior, and language processes. Knowledge itself serves no real purpose, at least none that is as worthwhile as the application of it to our personal and professional lives.

*Describe concepts or events in forms of specific operations performed.

SUGGESTED BIBLIOGRAPHY

Cathcart, Robert S. and Larry A. Samover: *Small Group Communication: A Reader*, 2d ed., Wm. C. Brown Co., Publishers, Dubuque, Iowa, 1974.

Condon, John C., Jr.: *Semantics and Communication*, 2d ed., Macmillan Publishing Co., New York, 1975.

DeVito, Joseph A.: *Language: Concepts and Processes*, Prentice-Hall, Englewood Cliffs, N.J., 1973.

ETC: A Review of General Semantics. The official organ of the International Society for General Semantics for the encouragement of scientific research and theoretical inquiry into nonaristotelian systems and general semantics (published four times a year).

General Semantics Bulletin, published by the Institute of General Semantics, which was founded in 1938 by Alfred Korzybski.

Glorfeld, Louis E.: *A Short Unit on General Semantics*, Glencoe Press (a division of the Macmillan Co.), New York, 1969.

Howe, Reuel L.: *The Miracle of Dialogue*, The Seabury Press, New York, 1963.

Krupar, Karen R.: *Communication Games*, The Free Press, New York, 1973.

Makay, John J. and Beverly A. Gaw: *Personal and Interpersonal Communication: Dialogue with the Self and with Others*, Charles E. Merrill Publishing Co., Columbus, Ohio, 1975.

Toffler, Alvin: *Future Shock*, Bantam Books, Inc., New York, 1970.

Watzlawick, Paul, Janet Helmick Beavin, and Don D. Jackson: *Pragmatics of Human Communication: A Study of Interactional Patterns, Pathologies, and Paradoxes*, W.W. Norton & Co., New York, 1967.

Part Two

Human Communication Concepts, Principles, and Methodologies Applied to Nursing

Communication is the lifeblood of our very being, the core of all human enterprise. The importance of communication in our lives as viewed by Thayer places it in good company. He said, "I would propose that communication be conceived as one of the two basic life processes—one being the acquisition and consumption of foodstuff for the organism's physical metabolism, or energy-processing; the other being the acquisition and consumption of physical and sensory event-data, or information processing."[1] The role of communication specifically in nursing is equally prestigious.

[1]Lee Thayer, "Human Communication: Tool, Game, Ecology," in Carl E. Larson and Frank E. X. Dance (eds.), *Perspectives on Communication,* Speech Communication Center, University of Wisconsin, Milwaukee, 1968, p. 13.

As I developed and wrote this manuscript, I was continuously questioning my boldness in entitling the book *Human Communication: The Matrix of Nursing*. I was going so far as to declare that communication was a part of not only *most,* but *all* nursing functions. At this point I believe I have convinced myself of that fact, and I hope sufficient evidence has been presented to convince the reader as well.

In this section, human communication concepts, principles, and methodologies presented in Part One will be applied to a number of functional areas of nursing. One separate chapter will be devoted to linking communication with each of the following areas: the nursing process, the nurse-client relationship, the teaching-learning process, management and change. In each of the five chapters, nursing students and registered nurses should be able to find material that is applicable to their activities whether their interest and/or position is in clinical practice, administration, or education. Most of the communication theory is equally applicable to all functional areas presented. However, to prevent *noise* from hitting your nervous system through redundancy, only a few relevant concepts or topics from Part I are presented under each chapter heading as a means of demonstrating how communication is involved.

While the parameters of nursing practice are continuously expanding and changing, there seems to be at least some agreement among nurses that nursing is a service of *helping people to help themselves in the area of health care*. It may be directed toward care required to attain greater physical and/or mental health or to maintain a maximum level of wellness or health. The responsibilities and activities of the nurse are related to helping the client cope with stress—stress related to (1) illness, its treatment, and/or efforts to maintain health; (2) changes required in one's life-style as a consequence of the disease, or illness and/or of the prescribed therapy or changes needed to maintain health; and (3) the environment in which health care is provided. While a degree of client dependence on the nurse may be acceptable at various stages in the caring process, the client's independence from health care providers, except for monitoring his health maintainence on a continuous basis, must be the ultimate goal of both the consumers and the providers of care. Communication skills in the hands of the nurse can facilitate that movement.

The nurse performs independent, dependent, and interdependent functions, each of which calls for a specific communication strategy. Nurses play the role of "client advocate," serving as client surrogate in communicating his requests and needs. Nursing activities in all areas of practice call for judgment, which relies upon our thought process, our intrapersonal communication skills, as well as our interpersonal communication ability when group decision making is required. Nurses' interpersonal communication skills are essential to successful functioning whether it is with clients, peers, the public, members of the health team, or personnel in other resource agencies. Nurses' responsibilities go beyond the confines of the health care agencies in which they are employed. Our ability to communicate effectively with government agencies and legislative bodies may be the critical variable in realizing our goal of quality health care for all people in our society. Only in recent years has the nursing population in general assumed its responsibility to speak out on health care issues.

Chapter 8

The Nursing Process

Nursing is the protection of the vulnerable.

Margaret Mead

From a human communication perspective, the *nursing process* can be viewed as the continuous gathering, processing, and utilizing of data related to the consumer's need for nursing care. It is generally outlined as a four-step process based on scientific problem-solving methods. As the basis for nursing practice, it becomes the concern not only of the nursing staff providing the direct care but of nursing administrative staff and educators as well. The steps in the process are (1) assessment of the client's needs for nursing care, (2) planning for the nursing care required, (3) implementation of the plan of care, and (4) evaluation of the care given. The process is a cyclic procedure whereby refinement and revisions in the plan and its initiation are made as the evaluation data dictate. All steps in the process of assessing, planning, implementing, and evaluating care depend strongly on the communication skills of the nurse.

STEPS IN THE PROCESS
Assessment

Nonverbal and verbal messages are received from a variety of sources and serve as the basis for identifying the nursing needs of each client. Some of the major sources of information are the admission record, which provides the demographic characteristics of the client, the medical history and examination, the client's record, planned and incidental observations, and formal interviews with the client and his family. Intuition remains a significant yet mystical source of information. In the area of psychiatric nursing, the mental status examination would of course provide valuable material. Clinical inferences are made by the nurse from the information available and are analyzed, synthesized, and interpreted in the form of nursing diagnoses.

Planning

A written nursing care plan is developed based on the assessment of client needs and can serve to provide continuity and consistency of care. Some knowledge of the client's frame of reference, learned from the assessment phase of the nursing process, should assist the nurse in suggesting potential alternatives available to the client as he copes with the stress experienced as the result of his illness. Preventive as well as therapeutic aspects of care are included in the plan. The client is actively involved in determining priorities of care and short- and long-term goals.

What is frequently missing in goal setting is establishing a specific period of time in which each particular goal can realistically be expected to be attained. The plan of care must contain a carefully plotted course, based on sequence in time, in the progression to the maximum level of independence. As more frequently happens in community health nursing than in hospital care, where limits are placed more rigidly on length of care, the same plan of care is used month after month with little concern for the time needed to attain certain levels of care. An alternative course of action might be long overdue. An interesting proposition by Grier[1] might be worthy of pursuing. She proposed that nurses be taught some decision-making theory so that the probabilities for favorable outcome could be considered in the decision-making process.

Intervention

Implementing the plan of care for meeting nursing needs entails a broad spectrum of nursing activities, all of which have a communication component. Vander Leest found that in her study of the nursing needs of clients in

---

[1]Margaret R. Grier, "Decision Making about Patient Care," *Nursing Research,* 25(2): 105–110, March-April 1976.

an ambulatory care center, those needs identified required primarily teaching and emotional support rather than technical care. The clients' lack of knowledge and understanding of their health problems was evident. From her findings she concluded that "The identification of and meeting of the major nursing needs of the ambulatory patient will require skill in communication."[2]

Reports and written records are the media used for communicating the client's clinical progress. The written records help to provide continuity of care and a progress report of the client. A potential value of the record which is often overlooked is as a data bank for clinical nursing research. The client's record also is required as legal documentation of the care given.

Among nurses the term *soaping* no longer relates only to the application of soap to a washcloth. It refers to a form of charting progress notes in structured but narrative form. Clients' problems are identified, and the nurse records the meaning of each problem as he or she views it in terms of subjective and objective data, assessment of the problem, and the proposed plan for resolving each problem. "S" refers to subjective data, such as an expressed symptom of dizziness by the client. "O" represents objective data, clinical findings, or observations by the nurse, such as pallor. "A" is the assessment that results from the analysis and synthesis of the data obtained from combining subjective and objective findings into a gestalt or calling to mind some condition of illness. "P" symbolizes the plan or proposed solution for the identified problem. As with the nursing process per se, the plan is based on a client-centered approach to care and upon the notion that the client is an active member of the health team. It therefore follows that the plan generally indentifies the responsibility to be assumed by the client as well as that to be assumed by the nurse. This type of charting represents an attempt to provide more relevant information as well as to weed out biases and inferences as much as possible.

Evaluation

Because communication is such an essential part of the nursing process, the evaluation results of the process might also be interpreted as an index of the communication effectiveness of the nurse. However, few valid tools are available for adequately evaluating the outcome of nursing intervention. Increasing numbers of instruments have been developed to evaluate the quality of nursing care, but they do not directly provide an answer to effective outcome. One of the more recently developed quality instruments was developed by researchers at Rush-Presbyterian-St. Luke's Medical

---

[2]Patricia A. Vander Leest, "The Nursing Needs of the Ambulatory Patient: Implications for Baccalaureate Programs in Nursing," unpublished doctoral dissertation, University of Denver, Denver, Colo., 1970, p. 118.

Center together with others from the Medicus Corporation. While their Quality Monitoring Tool does not reveal findings directly related to client welfare, studies have shown a positive relation between client outcomes and the quality of nursing care.[3] Nursing audits, using the records of discharged clients, have also been used to evaluate nursing care. The point remains that until adequate evaluating tools are developed, we will know little about the actual affect of health care in general on client outcome and the contribution made by nursing care per se.

In all four steps of the nursing process, the nurse is continuously serving as a communication center, receiving and sending messages. The vital inputs from the client, his family, observation, and all other information sources are carefully perceived, analyzed, synthesized, and interpreted by the nurse as to the meaning they have for him or her as he or she develops the plan of care.

THE CLIENT INTERVIEW

The most important source of information used in assessing client needs in the planning and provision of nursing care is the client interview. It requires a healthy relationship between the nurse (interviewer) and the client (interviewee), a psychological climate of trust and openness. If inaccurate and incomplete information is collected, an inaccurate nursing diagnosis will be made and inappropriate planning and intervention will be the result. Because of the importance of the data obtained from the client interview, the interview should remain an exclusive function of the professional nurse.

The conditions of the interview and purposes it serves are analogous to those of the counseling process. Both serve to (1) get information, (2) give information, and (3) establish a relationship or make a friend. The questions asked may themselves provide information to the client, as well as the client's response to the questions supplying information to the nurse. Data are gathered from verbal and nonverbal language of both parties, as both are actively involved in the process. Facial expressions, posture, general appearance, and personal hygiene all provide important messages.

The *quality and structuring of questions* directly affects the quality of the response. It should go without saying that the questions asked in the interview are based on the kinds of information required to determine the client's needs for nursing care. As with the counselor, the nurse interviewer should use an approach that is comfortable for him or her. One may

[3]Dieter Haussman, Sue Hegyvary, and John F. Newman, Jr., *Monitoring Quality of Nursing Care, Part II–Assessment and Study of Correlates,* HEW Publication No. (HRA) 76-7, July 1976.

prefer to use a highly *structured and written questionnaire* while another performs better with an *informal, free-flowing, spontaneous method of questioning*. There are obvious advantages and disadvantages to both. A highly formalized approach may retard the establishment of a healthy relationship, which situation in turn would be reflected in the quality of the information obtained. A more flexible, informal method would provide both individuals the opportunity to change the focus of the questioning in the direction that is most comfortable to them. For example, as questions of a more intimate nature were asked, a good interviewer would be perceptive of cues that indicated that the topic was too painful for the client to discuss at that time. The nurse would temporarily drop that area of questioning. Someone who was relying on a heavily structured questioning format might be less likely to deviate from it. Obviously there is less likelihood of needed information being missed with the structured interview.

There are a large number of classifications of categories of nursing needs that have been developed. They range in number of categories from a few to 21 or more. The five categories of needs identified by Fry[4] are all-inclusive and yet few in number, so that they can be recalled without the need for using written forms in the interview.

Another decision must be made regarding the recording of responses to the questions. Note taking during the session may not only be distracting but also encourage the client to conceal information. The task of remembering the responses and recording them after the interviewing process imposes the problem of accuracy. There may be a tendency to interpret the responses rather than objectively record them and to fill in the voids when information that was given cannot be recalled.

The *sequencing and wording of the questions* are important factors to consider. Each question should bear some logical relationship to the preceding question, thereby allowing the client to focus exclusively and completely on one subject area at a time. The more general questions will be followed by the more specific and intimate ones at a time when greater rapport should have been established. Because illness or the threat of illness tends to make individuals more egocentric, all questions should *first focus on the client* before going into family history and other areas of concern. Careful *pacing* of questions is essential so as to allow the client and nurse time to think about and recall information.

The judicious use of *silence and pauses* is recommended. Studies have revealed that the professional talks disproportionately more than the client. A change in this communication behavior might occur if the nurse got into the habit of periodically asking the client if he had any questions or recalled

[4]Vera Fry, "The Creative Approach to Nursing," *American Journal of Nursing,* 53(3): 301–302, March 1953.

additional information he had previously forgotten. At times an appropriately placed pause or period of silence may motivate the client to talk. Many individuals talk to relieve the discomfort they feel with silence. Again, the appropriateness of the silence rests largely with the nurse's *sensitivity to feedback* from the client.

An early clarification of the *terms of the communication contract,* including the purpose, roles expected of each member, and time limits, is advisable. In addition to the nurse tuning in to the client's feelings, the nurse must also be aware of messages unconsciously being sent to the client through nonverbal responses to his remarks. The *tone of voice* of both the nurse and the client affects the interpretation of the spoken words. For example, the nurse may verbally suggest a number of alternatives, but the tone of voice may clearly dictate to the client the choice to be made. *Double binds* should be identified by the nurse, called to the attention of the client, and clarified as to which message to follow.

Open-ended questions allow more freedom of response and provide more information, but are time-consuming. Each interview will be unique in part, because some clients are spontaneous in revealing the needed information while others reveal virtually nothing unless asked very specific questions and prodded for answers. Questions relating to *information that is already available from other sources* should be omitted unless there is some question of the validity and reliability of previous answers to those questions. Some *redundancy* in stating the questions is appropriate in efforts to clarify them to the client. The client should be able to expect the nurse to give her *undivided attention. External noise and interruptions* during the interview should be discouraged.

Sensitivity to cues is an art in itself. Cues are gained overtly from words uttered and covertly in patterned changes in overt topics, variations in voice quality, silence, things left unsaid or actions expected but not taken, and other nonverbal language

The client's *right of confidentiality* of conversation and medical records is generally a term of his Bill of Rights. However, it may be helpful for the nurse to reassure the client of how and where the information will be used. The nurse enters into an intimate relationship with the client, who is vulnerable and takes risks in revealing information of a very personal nature. The nurse must respect the trust placed in him or her and not violate that trust.

The information obtained from the interview should contain a clear and concise statement by the client of *his chief complaint.* What does the client himself perceive as his greatest distress and how does he think it might be alleviated? Too often the assessed client needs reflect what the *nurse* thinks the client needs should be or is a statement of a medical diagnosis. The nursing process must be client-centered, not staff-oriented. The client cannot be expected to respond to care based on what is not a true reflection of *his* needs. An interesting parallel might be drawn between our sensing something "unusual" happening in our body processes and some "unusual" behavior of our car. The consumer (client) should be in the best position to know and describe the problem and to some degree suggest ways the malady might be remedied, for he has lived closest and longest both with his car and his body. Mechanics and health professionals, who probably pride themselves on their expert judgment and knowledge, would do well to humble themselves and consider the suggestions of the experiencing consumer.

The client should also be questioned about his *expectations* of care and the role he is expected to play in the care, as well as his perceptions of his illness. Misconceptions can then be quickly corrected. He may be set to play the client role based on past personal experience with illness, from what neighbors and others have told him to expect, or from what he has experienced vicariously through television.

The *spatial-temporal dimensions* enter into the interviewing process in a number of ways. Because the data obtained in the interview are essential to the whole nursing process, they should be obtained as early as possible. *Timing* is especially important because doctors and others will or have already questioned the client. A lengthy interview may jeopardize the relevancy and accuracy of the data obtained. Vander Leest[5] found in her pilot study of twelve ambulatory care clinic clients that an average of 45 minutes was required for each interview using the structured guide relating to activities of daily living developed by Schwartz et al.[6] Again the nurse must be sensitive to feedback from the client and periodically inquire whether the client prefers to rest and resume questioning at another time.

The *spatial relation* of the nurse to the client is important because it dictates in part the type of relationship. If the nurse stands at the bedside of a reclining client, a physical and a possibly psychological one-upmanship relationship appears to exist. Conversely, if both parties are on the same physical plane, the important eye-to-eye contact will help convey a symmetrical relationship or a closeness between the individuals. Communication patterns will be established by the perceived relationship between members of the dyad.

The *states of both the nurse and the client* affect the communication behavior displayed in the interview. The nurse's theoretical knowledge, value system, priorities, and philosophy of nursing care will determine the line of questioning. It takes skill to refrain from communicating a judging attitude. The nurse must be objective and open to take in and process data that may seem impossible and unbelievable.

The client who is experiencing ill health or the threat of illness displays

[5] Vander Leest, "Nursing Needs of the Ambulatory Patient," p. 52.
[6] Doris Schwartz, Barbara Henley, and Leonard Zeitz, *The Elderly Ambulatory Patient: Nursing and Psychosocial Needs,* Macmillan Co., New York, 1964.

communication behavior that is different from that which the same person would exhibit if in good health. Physical impairment, for example, affects one's self-image, which in turn affects intrapersonal and interpersonal communication.

The person who is ill is more egocentric and more sensitive to his environment and to nonverbal communication than the well person. He is more imaginative in his perception of cues and meanings of words and responds more aggressively because of the threats to his security and life. He is more inclined to fill voids with self-referring meaning. He is more sensitive to his deep-level needs than normally and is concerned with fear of loss. Hearing acuity increases when an individual is under the stresses associated with illness, and thus he increasingly tries to refer what is said to himself. For example, if the staff is on rounds and is talking about a health condition in general that is totally unrelated to him, the client is inclined to twist the conversation to make sense as applying to him. The sense of touch is also heightened with illness.

The person who is ill searches very hard for structure in *what is said, what is observed,* and *what is not said or seen.* The voids, pauses, and silences take on important meaning to the ill individual. The client who is having his first experience with illness and the health care setting is usually searching diligently for cues. Misunderstanding and misevaluations result as he fills voids and responds to his own inputs. The ill individual is inclined to "read between the lines."

Illness behavior represents a coping response to difficulties of the situation. The client's tone of voice is a good indication of the urgency of the message. When a client says "I feel bad," there may be a message behind it which reads "Feel sorry for me" or "Do something about it." The physical and emotional disequilibrium associated with illness requires the nurse to use exceptional care in conveying messages to the client and his family, and in interpreting the meaning of messages from them.

HELPING THE CLIENT COPE

It is the responsibility of the nurse to assist the vulnerable to cope with the stresses in the area of health care. Communication again becomes that essential factor in helping the client successfully deal with the health problems confronting him. The most significant stresses in life are those imposed by other people and their social institutions.

1 *Helping the client cope with his illness, the prescribed therapy, and/or efforts to maintain health.* Through dialogue with the client, the nurse may be able to identify coping mechanisms the client has used

successfully in the past to deal with other stresses in life. The nurse can use communication skills to influence the client to again mobilize those forces within himself to deal with the stresses associated with his illness and its treatment. Efforts to maintain a high level of wellness, even without the experience of illness, can be equally distressing.

Some assistance may be provided as the nurse helps the client gain insight into his present experience of illness and his understanding of his behavior and reactions to stress. The nurse must interpret his *acting out* as his way of communicating hostility toward the illness and all it is perceived to mean in terms of loss.

Providing the client with information about his condition and its treatment may remove some misconceptions, reduce the unknown that is often the basis for fears, and help the client to make appropriate decisions. Very little in life is to be feared if it is understood.

The stress may be compounded if the client is not aware of the many alternatives or choices that may be available to him. The client may need to be moved away from the traditional either/or approach to coping. One is reminded of the delightful entertainer Maurice Chevalier, who on his 80th birthday was asked how he felt about getting old. His quick response was, "I didn't like the idea until I thought of the alternative." Too many people view illness as a threat or loss syndrome and not equally as a "win" alternative. The ill individual seldom is able to perceive the wealth of alternatives that may indeed be available to him. The nurse can help broaden his perspective.

During the client's illness, he must be kept actively involved in decision making throughout the total nursing process. He must be allowed to be in control, to make decisions that affect his life. Today laws are being written to help preserve that right. Prather put it clearly when he said: "I strongly object to the way elderly people are shoved around 'for their own good.' My grandmother has diabetes, and if knowing this she chooses to eat chocolates, that is her business. I would rather die in one year of candy than in ten of being watched over."[7] The nurse must examine her own values on this matter and the ways in which she communicates her beliefs to the client.

To develop a good *self*-support system, the client needs at least temporary support from others. The nurse should identify at least one family member who has the strength and ability to serve in that capacity. The nurse then should guide that individual in helping the client cope.

The nurse may be able to help the client identify the threat that is making him angry and anxious and express it openly so that he can more easily deal with it. Americans generally are proud of the right to say what they please, but in so many cases need help in getting the courage to say it.

The client's inability to cope with his illness may be perpetuated by his own behavior and compounded by those intimately involved with him: his family, the nursing staff, and other health professionals. While the goal of

[7]Prather, *I Touch the Earth, the Earth Touches Me*.

nursing care may be to help the client maintain his independence, stay in control, studies have shown that in actuality there is little reinforcement given to clients to encourage that kind of behavior. There is a tendency instead for the nurse to communicate and reinforce *dependent* behavior. The support of the nurse and others should be gradually but firmly withdrawn while confidence in the client's ability to handle his problems is communicated. The "pygmalion effect"[8] relates to the power to hinder or help the development of others through our expectations of them. Psychologists have demonstrated that the power of our expectations alone can influence others' behavior.

2 *Helping the client cope with changes required in life-style as a consequence of the illness, the prescribed therapy, or changes needed to maintain health.* "Man spends his life reasoning on the past, complaining of the present, and trembling for the future" and, one might add, especially trembling for a future that requires learning and adjusting to a new life-style. Coping with changes in one's life-style is not easy at any age.

It is helpful to identify the stresses that the client is experiencing early and help him resolve each one as it comes. The biographical sketch of the client gathered through the client interview provides a basis on which to study aspects of his past life-style that may need to change. The adage "You never puncture one part of the body without affecting other parts" is similar to Lewin's field theory and notion of *life space:* both relate to one's life-style. The individual can accommodate some changes in his life space, but when they are too many or come too fast the stress may be more than he can tolerate.[9]

The fact that illness frequently does require changes in one's life-style is supported by the findings of Vander Leest's study of ambulatory clinic clients. She found that 64 of the 100 clients interviewed believed their illness had changed their daily lives and 47 of that number considered that the changes required were major ones.[10]

The nurse must help restore the client's spirit and help him accept a new life-style that is more in concert with his physical and/or psychological abilities. The client must resolve the common conflict between what he wants to do and what it is possible for him to do. The nurse can provide the communication link between needed community services and the client. In some cases, a psychiatrist and other health care experts may need to be called in to help the client face reality.

In a sense the members of client's family are also clients. Their life-style will also be affected in one way or another. The nurse can provide them with support and information and serve in a preventive role by encouraging them to express their feelings.

[8]Robert Rosenthal, "The Pygmalion Effect Lives," *Psychology Today,* September 1973, pp. 56–63.
[9]Kurt Lewin, *Field Theory in Social Science: Selected Theoretical Papers,* Harper & Row, Publishers, New York, 1951, p. 25.
[10]Vander Leest, "Nursing Needs of the Ambulatory Patient," p. 75.

3 *Helping the client cope with the environment in which health care is provided.* The potential stress factors in our health care delivery system are legion. There are physical stressors in the environment and human-created stressors—the human-induced rules and policies of the institution, clinic, or agency. Any health care provider who cannot identify at least some of them has his head in the sand. Many of the problems are being made known as clients become more knowledgeable about the Bill of Rights. In fact, a man whose wife died of cancer in a large metropolitan hospital used a little-known and never-before used state statute to press for an investigation in which he contested the relicensure of that institution. In essence his complaint focused on his inability to get information from nurses, doctors, and other hospital personnel regarding his wife's care. In this case a family member was not trying to get financial redress but rather to press for the health care providers to assume their responsibility in communicating with families and clients. The man hoped that his action would prevent other families from experiencing similar problems and frustrations from the health care environment.

Many of the items that have been written into health care agencies' Patients' Bill of Rights,* especially those relating to the nonverbal language of time and space, relate to environmental factors. They include such rules as "the basic right to a human psychological and physical environment," "the right to have individual storage space for private use," "the right to privacy in dressing, toileting, and bathing," and "the right to receive visitors." It is a sad reflection on the nursing profession and other health care disciplines that these kinds of written requirements have ever had to been developed and enforced through legal action. Nurses now have not only the same responsibility they have always had in caring for clients but also the authority to see that a therapeutic environment be provided for every client with whom they come in contact.

Nurses must force themselves to be aware of the dangers that result from a client having to internalize hostility resulting from experiences he is having with dysfunctional factors in the environment in which he is receiving care. It makes little difference whether the hostility is due to being stripped of his identity as a hospitalized client or being forced to wait for appointed visits to a clinic. On more occasions than they realize, nurses are in a position to manipulate environmental factors to eliminate their detrimental effects. In other cases they may need to refer the matter to administrators or the proper authorities. The person who is ill is extremely sensitive to his environment, and nurses must be aware of ways by which they can structure his environment so that it will facilitate rather than impede recovery.

A few of the more glaring environmental stresses are presented here with some examples of how nurses have successfully eliminated them.

*The Medicare and Medicaid laws, Titles 18 and 19, respectively, require health care facilities receiving federal funds to have a written document outlining specific rights of the patients. The patients' Bill of Rights must be provided to each patient or his sponsor on admission to the facility. Additionally, federal law requires that all personnel in the facility receive training in implementation of the bill.

Why is it so often the case that the nurse on the hospital unit has little control over the assignment of clients to rooms and room assignment is based on a capricious decision from personnel in the admitting office? Roommate incompatability is stress-producing even when one is experiencing good health. Why aren't the assigned space and equipment of the client respected? Discourteous intrusion by personnel should not be condoned. Bed A and bed B are territorial labels, yet there is blatant violation of the client's right of possession. A study by Allekian[11] demonstrated that clients did indeed experience feelings of anxiety when their territorial domain in the hospital setting was invaded by hospital personnel.

Curtains are generally found dividing space in semiprivate rooms. Pulling them back without asking the client is an invasion of his territorial claim. In one community health nursing clinic, a nurse was able to replace the cloth cubicle curtains with more solid dividers. Clients were less reluctant to return for pap smears after that environmental change had been made.

Noise, primarily from staff, has been an eternal source of irritation. The use of the intercom system is an impersonal intrusion into one's private space. The "Quiet Please" and "No Smoking" signs seem only to apply to the minority: the clients and their families!

Outdated and unrealistic rules continue to pervade our health care facilities. In some places, husbands are still pleading to be allowed to attend deliveries or to visit their wife and newborn child in the hospital. The dearth of visitor lounges and other accommodations for families communicates only tolerance of families instead of an invitation for them to be a part of the plan of care.

The nurse *can* manipulate the environment in an effort to help the client cope with its stresses. The trainstyle arrangement of chairs in waiting rooms *can* be changed to provide a more social setting. Placing nursing home residents in wheelchairs in a circle, rather than in a line as if they were about to begin a race, *can* foster more communication among them.

The distressing fact of the waiting has already been discussed. If the waiting cannot be eliminated, why not have films available and provide public education to ease the discomfort of the wait? Dr. Middleton, a truly humanitarian physician who abhorred the impersonal nature of health care and the injustices to human worth and dignity, labeled the wait a "patent fault."[12] He went on to proclaim that "Medicine exists for the benefit of the afflicted and not the afflicted for the benefit of medicine." "Let's give the hospital back to the patients!" he exclaimed.[13]

Why do nurses persist with the untruth: "The doctor will be here in a

[11]Constance I. Allekian, "Intrusions of Territory and Personal Space: An Anxiety-Inducing Factor for Hospitalized Persons—An Exploratory Study," *Nursing Research,* 22(3):236–241, May–June 1973.
[12]William Shainline Middleton, *Values in Modern Medicine,* University of Wisconsin Press, Madison, 1972, p. 250.
[13]Middleton, *Values in Modern Medicine,* p. 251.

minute" or "I will be right back." To paraphrase A. Warwick, it is far better to do and not promise than to promise and not do. Even during hospitalization the client is forced to change a life-style of eating habits. Where are the clocks and calendars to keep individuals oriented to time? Even ecological guidelines are missing from hospital rooms without windows.

There are also numerous environmental stresses for the nurse which can be reflected in the quality of care given. A nurse worked in a very small outpatient examining room and was frustrated when, every step she took, she bumped into a piece of furniture. She counted 24 chair, table, desk, and equipment legs in that small room. She was able to remove some of the furniture, and a carpenter made several wall desks and tables without legs in the room. Her stress was reduced in half, for now she had to cope with only 12 furniture legs and her sense of crowding disappeared.

Nurses must be continuously on the alert for potential and existing stresses that the client himself might generate or that might emerge from sources external to himself. Nurses must use their creative ability and communication skills to help the client cope with these factors of stress.

SUGGESTED BIBLIOGRAPHY

Hammond, Kenneth, Katherine Kelly, Robert Schneider, and Margaret Vancini: "Clinical Inference in Nursing: Information Units Used," *Nursing Research,* 15(3): 236–243, Summer 1966.
———— and John Castellan, Jr.: "Clinical Inference in Nursing: Use of Information Seeking Strategies by Nurses," *Nursing Research,* 15(4):330–366, Fall 1966.
Kahn, Arlene Miller: "Relationship between Nurses' Opinions about Mental Illness and Experience," *Nursing Research,* 25(2):136–140, March-April 1976.
Katz, Violet: "Auditory Stimulation and Developmental Behavior of the Premature Infant," *Nursing Research,* May-June 1971, pp. 196–201.
Little, Dolores E. and Doris L. Carnevali: *Nursing Care Planning,* 2d ed., J. B. Lippincott Co., Philadelphia, 1976.
Marriner, Ann: *The Nursing Process: A Scientific Approach to Nursing Care,* C. V. Mosby Co., St. Louis, 1975.
Rush-Presbyterian-St. Luke's Medical Center and Medicus Systems Corporation: *Quality of Nursing Care: Assessment and Correlates,* Nursing Research Branch, Division of Nursing, February 1975.
Saxton, Dolores and Patricia A. Hyland: *Planning and Implementing Nursing Intervention,* C. V. Mosby Co., St. Louis, 1975.
Skipper, James K., Jr., Daisy L. Taliacozzo, and Hans O. Mauksch: "What Communication Means to Patients," *American Journal of Nursing,* 64(4): 101–103, April 1964.
Vander Leest, Patricia A.: *The Nursing Needs of the Ambulatory Patient: Implications for Baccalaureate Programs in Nursing,* unpublished Doctoral Dissertation, University of Denver, Denver, Colo, 1970.

Chapter 9

The Nurse-Client Relationship

When love and skill work together expect a masterpiece.

Ruskin

Nursing is a social process in which there is an *intimate* relationship between the nurse and the client. The relationship is contiguous with every nursing function, whether it be providing physical, emotional, or supportive care or getting information from or supplying information to the client in an effort to help him care for himself and his illness. A *therapeutic* relationship is one in which the psychological climate is such that it facilitates positive change and growth in the client. The *therapeutic use of self,* formerly considered to be the unique tool of the psychiatric nurse, is now viewed as a necessary part of the professional paraphernalia of all nurses irrespective of their area of practice.

THE NURSING LITERATURE

Nurses are often glib as they talk about establishing therapeutic relations with the clients. But upon being questioned about what they mean by "therapeutic" relations, what conditions are needed to attain them, and how they evaluate their presence, they often are at a loss to reply. The nursing literature is saturated with isolated factors relating to the nurse-client relationship, but few instances are found in which all of the needed conditions are presented and operationally defined so that tools can be developed to assess the effectiveness of the relationship. The fact that communication skills are involved is evident by the direction taken in some of the research studies. The verbal-behavior characteristics of the nurse and client have been studied in terms of message content, task and process functions, and the number of verbal utterances made by both parties in the relationship. Audio and/or video tape recordings, transcripts, and process records have all served as data for study of the interpersonal phenomenon. Some interaction researchers have used physiological measures as criteria variables. For example, Foster[1] used a measure of adrenal activity to study the association between stress and the nurse-client relationship. She hypothesized that reduction in stress through interpersonal communication would be reflected in reduced adrenocorticotrophic hormone output. Using urinary sodium/potassium ratio as an adrenal cortex stress indicator, she concluded that it was a valid index of the body's biochemical response to stress and thus a reflection of client welfare.

The nursing literature supports the idea that the nurse must be genuine and open in the relationship with the client. If the nurse enters the relationship as a person rather than a technician or a nurse, the client is more inclined to be himself. Yet stereotypes continuously portray the nurse as a rigid professional lacking in spontaneity and openness. Undoubtedly the professional attire of many nurses continues to perpetuate this undesirable stereotype. The masks nurses wear in the operating rooms are insignificant compared with the masks they hide behind when relating to clients.

Nurses are encouraged to accept people as they are, to be nonjudgmental as they assist the clients in times of stress. If the client is to be free to express himself, the nurse must be approachable, accepting, flexible, and tolerant and communicate that in their encounters. The client must perceive the interest, caring, and trust offered by the nurse. van Kaam[2] summarized the quality of a therapeutic relationship as one in which the client has a need to be understood. He feels he is understood when he can *sense* the nurse's understanding and when the nurse, as a person, coexperiences what the illness means to the client and continues to accept him.

[1]Sue B. Foster, "An Adrenal Measure for Evaluating Nursing Effectiveness," *Nursing Research,* **23**(2):118–124, March-April 1974.
[2]Adrian L. van Kaam, "The Nurse in the Patient's World," *American Journal of Nursing* **59**:1708–1710, 1959.

ROGERS'S APPROACH TO THE THERAPEUTIC RELATIONSHIP

The philosophy, concepts, and desired outcomes generally presented in the nursing literature relating to the nurse-client relationship are in concert with those identified, described, and tested by Carl Rogers.[3] He described a therapeutic relationship as one in which (1) two individuals are in psychological contact, (2) the client is in a state of incongruence, being vulnerable or anxious, (3) the therapist is *congruent, or genuine,* in the relationship, (4) the therapist experiences *unconditional positive regard* for the client, (5) the therapist experiences *empathic understanding, or accurate empathy,* of the client's frame of reference, and (6) the therapist's attitudinal conditions are *communicated to* and *perceived by* the client at least to a minimal degree.

Rogers, the "father" of nondirective, or client-centered, counseling,[4] theorized that it is not what one does but *how* one does it in the relationship that provides the therapeutic conditions antecedent to change. The three interpersonal qualities of the therapist of accurate empathy, congruence, and unconditional positive regard are *attitudes* and are not identified as specific behaviors. It follows that they must to be *learned experientially* and not intellectually.

Rogers defined *accurate empathy* as the therapist's understanding of the client's feelings and ability to sense the private world of the client *as if* it were his own—as the ability to "walk in his shoes." Empathic individuals generally are considerate of others and do not make rash judgments. Females have been found to be more interpersonnally aware than males. To be sensitive to others requires insight into self and openness. Empathy is a difficult concept to study in our interpersonal communication. However, there is strong research evidence that having a high degree of empathic understanding makes one a better nurse, teacher, counselor, and parent.

A therapist who is *congruent* is genuine and open, neither denying nor withholding his own feelings from the client. It is important that there be a person-to-person, not a nurse-to-client, relationship in the sense of the nurse acting in a sheltered professional role. The other two conditions of empathy and personal regard are also enhanced when the client views the nurse as human. The need to be real and sincere reminds the author of the story of a stone carver who was to display his works at an art show. As he was putting some finishing touches to the man he had carved out of stone, he accidentally chipped off one of the arms. The judges would soon appear to judge his work. Time was at a premium. It was suggested that he leave the

[3]Carl R. Rogers, "The Necessary and Sufficient Conditions of Therapeutic Personality Change," *Journal of Consulting Psychology,* 21:95–103, 1957.
[4]Carl R. Rogers, *Client-Centered Therapy: Its Current Practice, Implications, and Theory,* Houghton Mifflin Co. Boston, 1951.

arm off. Another suggestion was that he quickly mold the arm out of wax. The stone carver decided on that idea and proceeded to make the arm, which was nearly perfect and did not look like what it really was. As the judges came down the line of carvings, the sun shone in from a nearby window and the wax hand melted away. The stone carver was quickly excluded from the judging, for his sculpture was not *sincere*—not "without wax." Nurses, also, must guard against falsifying their true being, or they, too, will be judged harshly by the clients they are trying to help.

The third attitudinal condition needed for establishing and maintaining a therapeutic relationship is *unconditional positive regard*. This phrase describes a therapist who provides a warm, permissive, nonthreatening atmosphere in the encounter. The therapist demonstrates an unconditional acceptance and a caring for the client which is nonpossessive in character. Howe[5] also considered abnormal dependence or possessiveness of one member of the dyad toward the other as impairing the relationship and dialogue.

In addition to the therapist's triad of conditions being present in the relationship, the client must *perceive* these therapist-offered attitudes at least to a minimal degree, according to Rogers. In other words, the therapist must provide the kinds of messages that will help convey his attitudes so that they will be perceived as such by the client. In order for behavior to change, a change in perception must be experienced.

Each of the conditions exists along a continuum. Rogers theorized that the greater the degree to which these conditions are present in the relationship, the greater the chances of constructive personality and behavioral changes in the client. Some study findings have substantiated the relationship between presence of the conditions and constructive outcome.

The task of developing research instruments to test Rogers's theory was not an easy one. It required tools for measuring intangibles in a situation filled with fluid subtleties. However, he and his associates constructed a Condition Scale for each of the three attitudinal conditions. The research design using these scales and the findings appear in the book Rogers edited relating to psychotherapy with schizophrenics.[6]

RESEARCH FINDINGS ON THE NURSE-CLIENT RELATIONSHIP

Rogers had proposed that the conditions of a therapeutic relationship were appropriate to the study of any interpersonal relationship in a helping situation. Nursing, in which relationships are established as the nurse helps

---

[5]Howe, *The Miracle of Dialogue*, p. 68.
[6]Carl R. Rogers, (ed.) *The Therapeutic Relationship and Its Impact: A Study of Psychotherapy with Schizophrenics*, University of Wisconsin Press, Madison, 1967.

the client cope with stress, was considered to be an appropriate field for study. Using Rogers's theoretical model, a research study was conducted of the nurse-client relationship in the home setting.[7] Thirty nurse-client dyads served as subjects. The clients ranged in age from 17 to 91. The entire nursing visit in each of the client sample homes was tape-recorded. The visits ranged in length from 11 to 70 minutes. The 30 visits produced a total of 16.8 hours of recorded nurse-client interaction.

Nine judges were trained in the three attitudinal conditions of empathy, congruence, and unconditional positive regard. They then listened to two 3-minute systematically obtained segments of the total interaction of each visit and rated each relationship using the Condition Scales of Rogers. In addition, a 64-item self-report questionnaire was completed by each of the 30 nurses and clients and by all 9 judges. The questionnaire was the Barrett-Lennard Relationship Inventory, which was also patterned after Roger's theory of a therapeutic relationship.[8] It provided the data needed to determine the degree to which the nurse had communicated the attitudinal conditions to the client and his perception of them.

Only 2 of the 30 nurses studied reached the level of attitudinal conditions prescribed as a therapeutic relation. Neither of these two nurses reached a maximum level of functioning in any of the three conditions. The clients, nurses, and judges all varied in their perception of the relationship as determined by their response to the Relationship Inventory. A score of 192 represented the best possible nurse-client relationship perceived. The average level of the relationships as perceived by the clients (137.6) was much higher than that perceived by the nurses (96.7) or the judges (62.9). It is not uncommon to find disparity in perceptions between clients and health care providers because each group has its own unique expectations of the relationship and of care.

Empathy, which is considered to be of utmost importance in providing nursing care, was judged to be at or above the midpoint on the Condition Scale for only four (13 percent) of the nurses studied. As rated by the judges, five nurses failed to function at the midpoint level on *any* of the three conditions. The findings failed to describe very successful relationships between the nurses and the clients.

The findings are discouraging especially when one considers the importance placed on establishing a therapeutic relationship and when the relationship is such an integral part of all nursing care. Some consolation may be gained from the findings of similar studies, which revealed that

[7]Margaret L. Pluckhan, "The Nurse-Patient Relationship in the Home Setting," unpublished doctoral dissertation, University of Denver, Denver, Colo., 1970.

[8]G. T. Barrett-Lennard, "Dimensions of Therapist Response as Casual Factors in Therapeutic Change," *Psychological Monographs: General and Applied,* **76**(43; whole no. 562), 1962.

counselors, psychologists, and psychiatrists also functioned at minimal or below minimal therapeutic levels.

According to Howe[9] abnormal dependence may get in the way of establishing a truly helping relationship. Kalisch[10] expressed her concern with nurses fostering dependency of the client rather than helping him to be free to develop and use his own self-support system. She questioned whether, through verbal and nonverbal influence when helping clients cope with stress, nurses might be controlling adult clients and casting them in such childlike ways as to foster dependency. Whatever the answer may be, further research study together with new approaches to improving nurses' ability to become more empathic, congruent, and accepting must be considered. Some of the training and practice suggested by Truax and Carkhuff[11] might be well to consider.

APPLICATION TO OTHER RELATIONSHIPS

All of what has been presented relating to the nurse-client relationship is equally applicable to the parent-child, teacher-student, or supervisor–staff nurse relationship. Emerson's words "A true friend is somebody who can make us do what we can" reflect the goal of a therapeutic relationship. It has been said that a person who pays a therapist is actually purchasing a friend. One need not be a professional to engage in therapy. Friends have most of the essential qualities needed in therapy, and they offer their services and help without charge. The relationship of nurses and doctors on the health team has additional factors of concern, not the least of these being the threat of territorial encroachment by one another. A major step toward improved relationship can come when we view the team in the equal portions of the pie rather a than hierarchical pyramid perspective.

SUGGESTED BIBLIOGRAPHY

Conant, Lucy H.: "Give-and-Take in Home Visits," *American Journal of Nursing,* **65**(7):117–120, 1965.
———, "Use of Bales' Interaction Process Analysis to Study Nurse-Patient Interaction," *Nursing Research,* **14:** 304–309, 1965.
Howe, Reuel L.:*The Miracle of Dialogue,* The Seabury Press, New York, 1963.
Johnson, Walter L. and Helen M. Simon: "Some Aspects of the Interaction of Public Health Nurses and Patients in Home Visits," *American Journal of Public Health,* **51:**95–105, 1961.

[9]Howe, *The Miracle of Dialogue* p. 68.
[10]Beatrice J. Kalisch, "An Experiment in the Development of Empathy in Nursing Students," *Nursing Research,* **20:**202–211, May–June 1971.
[11]Charles B. Truax and Robert R. Carkhuff, *Toward Effective Counseling and Psychotherapy: Training and Practice,* Aldine Publishing Co., Chicago, 1967.

Kiesler, Donald J., Philippa L. Mathieu, and Marjorie H. Klein: "Sampling from the Recorded Therapy Interview: A Comparative Study of Different Segment Lengths," *Journal of Consulting Psychology,* **28:**349–357, 1964.

Peitchinis, Jacquelyn A.: "Therapeutic Effectiveness of Counseling by Nursing Personnel: Review of the Literature," *Nursing Research,* **21:**138–148, March-April 1972.

Rogers, Carl R. and Barry Stevens: *Person to Person: The Problem of Being Human,* Real People Press, Lafayette, Calif., 1967.

Wallston, Kenneth A. and Barbara S. Wallston: "The Use of Simulated Nursing Unit to Investigate the Listening Behavior of Nurses to Patients," *Nursing Research,* **24:**16–22, January-February 1975.

Chapter 10

The Teaching-Learning Process

Observations more than books, experience rather than persons, are the prime educators.

A. B. Alcott

Prevention of illness and maintenance of health have taken on added importance in our health care delivery system. The increasing number of Health Maintenance Organizations (HMOs) is but one example. The nursing profession can pride itself on being ahead of the times in stressing prevention through *health teaching*. This has been particularly true in the field of community health.

Nurses are actively involved in the teaching-learning process in many ways other than client teaching and general public education. They are engaged as students and teachers in formal educational programs, in staff development and in-service education programs in the work setting, and in the all-important continuing education programs. *Continuing education* is rapidly moving from a voluntary to a mandatory basis of requiring health professionals and members of other disciplines to keep abreast of changes in their field of practice. The need for continuing education might be considered analogous to the fish market, where the need for constant renewal becomes obvious in a relatively short period of time.

Health education for the general public is directed toward mobilizing the public's self-help potential. The nurse can educate lay people to help themselves and others in need of physical and mental health care. It is reported, for example, that only about 12 percent of the people with mental health problems actually use mental health care facilities. Nurses are in a position to teach bartenders, beauticians, and other human service groups to serve in the capacity of "friend" and as a source of referral to health care agencies.

THE TEACHER-STUDENT RELATIONSHIP

The teacher has a responsibility to provide a climate conducive to learning, motivate the student, provoke thought, and serve as a model. The qualities of the nurse-client relationship, described in the previous chapter, are equally applicable to the teacher-student helping relationship. The teacher must have empathic understanding of the student's frame of reference and use that knowledge as a basis for the approach to transmitting the subject matter. It is obvious that if audience members are heterogeneous, with little in common in their backgrounds, adjusting the teaching approach to accommodate such a diverse membership will be difficult. To be congruent, or genuine, both parties must be at ease and comfortable in the situation and respond as people. Again, much can be lost if the teacher conveys a one-upmanship attitude to the students. The teacher may help communicate his or her humanness by revealing personal experiences that convey the message that "the leader of the flock is to be a sheep like all the rest." Unconditional positive regard is evident when students are not embarrassed to answer or ask questions, for example. The teacher communicates a high regard for their involvement, and no question is too unimportant or too ridiculous.

THE NURSE AS TEACHER

Many nurses remain convinced that client teaching is not *their* responsibility but that of the physician. Yet in a study conducted over a decade ago, it was found that the clients wanted to communicate with the nurse *to get information* as well as to make the day more pleasant through conversation. From the nurse's communication with them, they inferred that the nurse was dedicated, interested, and possessed of the technical competence, knowledge, and skill needed to get them well.[1] Vander Leest found that of 100 clients interviewed in an ambulatory care center, 50 percent said they had been told *little or nothing* by the doctor. The principal nursing intervention required, identified from client needs assessment, was found to be client teaching.[2]

Client teaching may be conducted on a one-to-one basis or in a group. The size of the group depends upon the *content* being presented and the *homogeneity* of the members. An obvious advantage to group learning experiences results from clients being allowed time to share their experiences and learn from one another as well as from the nurse. The *physical arrangement and setting* influence the free exchange of ideas. The *verbal language* used must be appropriate for all members of the group, and medical jargon should be used with discretion. *Redundancy* may be helpful, especially with a heterogeneous group. The selection of *media* is an important consideration. Many useful films are available from such agencies as the cancer, heart, and mental health associations. They can be used with individual or group teaching methods at the client's bedside, in classrooms, or in outpatient clinics. In all teaching-learning situations, the terms of the communication contract should be made clear at the start of all sessions.

THE CLIENT AS TEACHER

Probably in no other relationship is there such an opportunity for members of a dyad to exchange roles more readily than in the teaching-learning process involving the nurse and the client. Nurses, however, have been remiss in not fully utilizing the teaching potential of the client. Indeed, as Emerson said, "The secret of education lies in respecting the pupil." The nurse's textbook knowledge of response to illness is second-hand and inferential compared with the valuable first-hand and factual information available from the clients themselves. Client report is a clinically rich source of information with the potential of generating new insights for professionals to use in helping other clients cope —with illness and its therapy, with changes required in life-styles, and with the health care environment.

By way of example, the following is the actual account, presented exactly as it was written by Mr. Rodgers, of his experience with illness. As

[1]James K. Skipper, Jr., Daisy L. Tagliacozzo, and Hans O. Mauksch, "What Communication Means to Patients," *American Journal of Nursing,* **64**(4):101–103, April 1964.
[2]Vander Leest, "Nursing Needs of the Ambulatory Patient, p. 77.

you read his report, identify the sources of stress and consider ways in which a nurse might help him cope with them. There is a wealth of meaning in his messages which can serve as cues to the type of physical and emotional care a nurse could provide to help him through his experiences.

"I had that feeling that this wasn't really happening to me. I was some sort of an impersonal observer, but that poor unfortunate individual to whom it was happening was certainly in trouble. I think I knew, or at least had strong suspicions from the very beginning, what was wrong, but I had a hard time accepting it or that it was me to whom it was happening. Less than a month previously, my father had died of a coronary thrombosis. One of my best friends was recovering from one. Another had died a couple of months previously. So I was very conscious of the threat of the disease, and the symptoms were not particularly surprising to me.

This was a morning in mid-March, a better than average morning for me. There were optimistic financial prospects. Physically, I felt unusually well. I arose early (6:00 A.M.) and attended a chamber of commerce breakfast downtown. I had quite an appetite, and I remember I ate my food faster than I should have. Breakfast consisted of scrambled eggs, sausage, and toast, washed down with two cups of strong black coffee. There was a speaker. I listened attentively. The meeting was over at 8:30 — too early to complete the three errands I had downtown. So I killed time by walking around, I walked unhurriedly for about a mile. An attractive restaurant caught my eye. The atmosphere and a place to loaf appealed to me more than the need for nourishment. But I went on in after buying a morning paper, ordered a cinnamon roll and black coffee, and ate again just to be unobtrusive, while I broused through the paper. It was now nearly 9:30 — time to get busy. I still felt fine. I got up, paid my check, and left the restaurant. My manner now became purposeful. My pace had quickened. I strode along for about a block. In a matter of four steps, the whole damned world collapsed. I underwent a 'Dr. Jekyll and Mr. Hyde' change, for in rapid successive steps I went from that youthful feeling to a feeling of decandent old age. First, there was a sense of dizziness. It was quick and severe. I stopped in my tracks. The worst of it passed quickly, leaving me with a head that felt like a lump of coal and a completely confused mind. My arms and legs were heavy. When I began to walk again it was like struggling through a swamp of black, sucking mud. Actually, movement involved tremendous concentration. Sense of direction was all but destroyed. I broke out in a cold sweat, and it was then that I had the feeling described earlier in which I was a disinterested observer. Other people on the street seemed very distant and silent. I was not conscious of street noises at all. My throat was dry and constricted. Perhaps there was some pain even then, but I don't remember it. I was too busy trying to keep up with events as they happened.

What to do now? I was in front of another restaurant — perhaps a glass of water would help. I went in, found a stool at a nearby counter, and sat there stupidly. I worried a little about being taken for a 'drunk' and tried to snap myself out of it. I was successful to the extent of asking for the glass of water, but it was a great effort. Then I just sat and hoped. Sure enough, the condition began to pass. I promised myself to get in and get a physical checkup at the earliest possible opportunity, and I reassured myself that this really wasn't the real thing at all. 'After all, Rodgers, you're 46 years old. You gotta expect some growing pains, you know. Doctor will probably tell you to take off some weight again and that you're strong as a bull and full of the same, and that will be that.' I sat there for 20 minutes to half an hour. I felt strong enough to travel, confident, and clear-headed—well, almost. No one was probably giving me a second thought, but I was self-conscious, like the whole human race was centered on me—that people were looking at me—and that was making me uncomfortable. So I got up and paid my check. I had ordered a glass of milk which I didn't drink —just ordered it to keep from feeling conspicuous. It seemed to me that the cashier looked at me strangely. Maybe my color was a little green around the edges or something.

My car was parked two blocks away. A few minutes before I couldn't have told you where it was, but now I knew. I was a little more respectful of the situation. Was now imagining all sorts of things. I walked slower but without too much apprehension for about half the distance. Then the old feeling began to slowly return and persist until it was almost as bad as before, and I remember reflecting 'If it's gotten so bad in so short a time, will I still be among the living an hour from now?' then quickly rationalizing to myself: 'This could be the flu, you know; it's been doing some strange things this spring. If I could just get home and lie down for awhile. — Well, why not? Haven't got too much that has to be done this morning, anyway. I'll just run the one more errand and go home.

I finally reached the car and for the next half-hour just sat with my head on my arm on the steering wheel recuperating. 'What's the matter with you, Rodgers? You're certainly overdramatizing this thing,' I scolded. 'You've had pains before. This is just some small thing. Stomach's a little upset. Maybe it's a coffee jag. You drink too much too fast, and it makes you dizzy. You had three cups this morning already, you know. Better cut that down—join 'Coffee Anonymous' or something.' Then, as my head began to clear, 'Anyway, you feel better now; forget it.'

Sometime along about here, I was conscious of tingling numbness in my left arm and shoulder. There were dull chest pains with an occasional sharp jabbing one. But it wasn't the pain so much as an impending loss of consciousness, apprehension, the great effort required to perform the smallest of tasks, shortness of breath, heaviness of arms and legs, stomach upset, and that '90-year-old sensation.'

I started the car and headed out into traffic in the direction of my errand about four blocks away. 'What if I lose consciousness in this traffic? Not much chance of that. I've never been unconscious in my life except when asleep. Anyway, I couldn't stay there all day.'

Giddiness persisted. There were moments of downright dizziness that passed quickly, and there was that tingling in my left arm and that slight pain high on my left chest, like a muscular soreness that really told me the facts of life in spite of my stubborn rationalization. Then there were stabbing little pains in the center of my chest and in my back. But they weren't serious—the same sort of pains you experience heralding a chest cold coming on.

I had no trouble finding a parking place close to the entrance of the building I wanted to visit. It wasn't more than 200 feet to the door, but it seemed more like 20 miles of slogging mud. Inside the door was a straight chair. I couldn't get past it. But now I was conscious of another sensation. No matter whether I was sitting down or standing up, I wasn't comfortable. Sitting down, I wanted to be up. Standing up, I wanted to sit or lie down. So I didn't sit still long.

The man I had come to see had an office on the main floor. So I made my way back to his desk. His secretary told me he was out for coffee. I could join him, or he would be back in a few minutes. I declined the offer and seized the opportunity to again sit down — this time in his swivel chair, in which I leaned as far back as possible. I disciplined myself to sit still and in a few minutes was breathing a little easier. I don't know why I suddenly wanted to talk to my wife, Rilla, and tell her all about it. After all, the best that could do was make her worry. Must have been that 'Misery loves company.' Anyway I reached for the phone on the desk and dialed my home number. It was sure good to hear a friendly and concerned voice. I had never felt so alone in my life right in the middle of a teeming city. I told her that I didn't feel well and was coming home. Then I fixed things up swell by telling her that if I didn't arrive in a reasonable time she could start looking for me along West Colfax. That was very reassuring to her, but then, I was surely thinking of myself exclusively about then.

Rilla knows me. We've been married 23 years. She ought to. So she just pointed out that I always get excited at the first symptom—that I'm probably getting the flu—that I never take care of myself anyway, and that it could have even been something I ate like those link sausages. I wanted to believe that, but a disturbing voice within me had already warned, 'You're in trouble. You're really in trouble this time. . . .'

My business took less than 5 minutes when my man returned, and I didn't say one unnecessary word to prolong the conversation. It was exhausting exertion as it was. After I said goodbye, I headed back toward the front door. My throat was dry, and there was a peculiar, hard-to-describe, heavy feeling in my stomach or just above it. Back through my legs and arms crept that heaviness, and then there was that tingling left arm and the pains in chest and back.

'God,' I said to myself, 'I'll never get to that front door, let alone get home.' This time the sweating was more profuse. I unfastened my tie and collar. Huge beads of perspiration stood out on my forehead. 'Oh, God, don't let me drop here — let me get home. This must really be serious. Got to get fixed up. It's going to take time. Time I haven't got. There's that chair by the door. I'll keep my eye on that chair. Hope I make it. That chair is my only objective in life. If I can just make that chair, maybe I can get home.'

Strange, I hadn't thought of calling a doctor yet. 'Better not call yet. They hate to be bothered before office hours. Call after you get home,' had been the thought with which I dismissed that solution when the sensations first hit me an hour and a half before.

Now I began thinking again about calling a doctor. 'Which one should I call?' I had had a physical examination each year over a long period of time. Only thing they ever found was a little high blood pressure. I knew a dozen doctors in the city socially, but I couldn't think of a name (that old confusion again.) I couldn't even remember the name of our family doctor without great concentration. I finally remembered it and resolved to call him just as soon as I got near a phone. Now I noticed a marked sensation along my neck like a rope being drawn tight around it. In my mouth, my gums hurt where teeth had been extracted years before. Now I had to concentrate all my energy on maintaining a true course to that chair. 'Mustn't lose sight of it—might never be able to sight it again.' At last I could reach out and touch it. I had made it. Sitting on the chair, I gave up the idea of trying to find my way home unaided.

The chair was right beside a public telephone booth. I called Rilla again and told her that I wasn't going to be able to make it. She asked me if I had called the doctor. When I told her I hadn't, we decided that was the next thing to do. She said she would call her brother and ask him to come after me.

After the call I stepped out into the outer office. I was exhausted and feeling more uncomfortable than ever. It was a reception room with two or three chairs and a davenport so that I was able to half recline on the davenport. The wave did not pass this time, as it had done previously, and I abandoned my effort to act as if nothing was happening. I explained my situation as briefly as possible to the receptionist and asked her to phone my doctor. She soon reported that he was out and couldn't be reached until 2:30. I couldn't think of another doctor. I sank back and waited for my brother-in-law.

He wasn't long in coming. I walked out and climbed in his car. I remember wondering how many traffic tickets I would accumulate on my car parked where it was before I could get back to it again. He asked me where I wanted to go. I had visions of searching through office buildings for a doctor who could take the time to treat me. Finally I told him that I thought a hospital would be our best bet. He asked which one. I thought the closest one was the city hospital, and the closest one was the one I wanted right then.

The bed in the emergency ward surely looked good. I realized all the vital statistic questions they began plying me with were necessary, but they surely were exhausting. Then began the parade of interns, internists, doctors, and nurses of all descriptions. Each one asked the same questions over and over again. The doctor in the emergency ward gave me a quick examination. Said he thought I could go on home. Then somewhere in that maze of faces two appeared that became very familiar to me in the days immediately following. They ordered an electrocardiogram and later announced the diagnosis of coronary thrombosis and that I couldn't be moved from the hospital.

They wheeled me up on the ward, gave me a shot, and let me rest. I wasn't in any great pain, and as long as I laid still it felt good. About every so often, another guy in a white coat would stick his head around the corner and ask all the same questions again. I would rattle off my now memorized story as best as my drug-clouded mind could convey it, and he would disappear. After a while another would appear, etc.

The nurses and nurses aides were very solicitous, and all in all the afternoon passed quickly. My wife was allowed to sit with me. Along in the evening, the doctor brought a rubber hose connected to oxygen, which he announced he was going to run up my nose and down my throat. My nose was broken in high school football, and this project proved irritating, uncomfortable, and finally impossible. Within a few minutes they wheeled in oxygen equipment with a plastic tent, and I became one of the tent people.

There were a dozen other patients on the ward, most of whom I considered sicker than myself. The nurses were terribly rushed, and in my oxygen tent I felt cut off from the world. At first I experienced a degree of claustrophobia. The doctor emphasized that he wanted me to lie perfectly still in that the danger was extremely grave that I might have a second and more serious attack within the next few hours. This tied in with my recent experience with my father. He had one in the morning and the fatal one that evening. So I was properly scared stiff.

Sometime during that afternoon I met the attending specialist for the illness. On his first visit he described me as a slightly obese male. Funny, I had never considered myself 'obese.' True, I am 6 feet 1½ inches tall and at that time weighed from 205 to 207 pounds in my street clothes—but being pot-faced and round-bellied, I thought of myself as just arriving at a comfortably plump middleage. Though I had been knocking myself out trying to establish a profitable business, I was unaware of the extra burden of an extra 35 or 40 pounds excess weight that I was carrying around. Yes, I had business worries. Lots of them. I am what is classified in William H. Whyte's *Organization Man* as a 'middle management guy,' meaning that I get pressure from all sides, above, below, and horizontally from both sides. So that evening I was particularly worried about how the world was going to survive without the effort I was ordinarily expected to make in the next 48 to 56 hours. That's about how far ahead I was thinking, but I was suffering thinking about all the things I had left to the last minute that just weren't going to get done now—feeling sorry for myself about how close I had come to success before my strength failed. I certainly didn't consider myself in any critical danger. At that point I was already feeling good enough to pose that everlasting question, 'When am I going to get out of here?' How ignorant can you be? I hadn't even begun the fight yet, and I thought I really knew something about heart trouble.

The uncomplaining, quiet way the nurses accepted the trials and tribulations of waiting on the other patients in the ward inspired me to try and be as little trouble as I could, and I hope I succeeded. One thing that left me a little panicky was the fact that I didn't have a bell I could ring for a nurse, and I couldn't yell without discomfort. I couldn't move without assistance, or so I had been cautioned; yet if I needed more blanket or less or help with any of the bodily requirements, I had a great deal of trouble attracting enough attention to get them taken care of. I perfected a very satisfactory bellow in the weeks that followed, and I am sure I disturbed the patients around me just as much as they disturbed me during the first few days of my hospital confinement.

The food was not to my taste, and my doctors didn't care a bit. It would be nice if everybody who prescribes diets would live on them for at least a week sometime. However, perhaps my doctors did, for they were most sympathetic, but each tray contained the same LePages Glue, water, and sawdust (that's what it tasted like). Let me hasten to say that this is not the dietician's fault. I realize she cooks according to the requirements laid down by the doctors. But anyway the lack of seasoning made all kinds of meat, vegetable, and fruit taste just alike.

Anyway, going back to the first day. In the evening the doctor drew the first blood I remember for the prothrombin time. Then all night long he kept checking it. He didn't say much, was very methodical and matter-of-fact. I tried to wisecrack a little, I guess to bolster my courage, but it didn't go over with him. He told me what he thought I should know and answered my questions as carefully and patiently as he possibly could, and there our verbal relationship ended. But when it came to performance, he couldn't do enough for me. And the way he worked over me was most reassuring. I am sure he and the other doctors contributed a great deal to the rapidity of my convalescence.

The days melted one into another. I became reconciled to the fact that this was no 2- or 3-day illness. My worst concern now was dread of the bedpan ordeal and my bedsoreness and weariness. There were no bedsores from lack of nursing care. Rather it was the bonesoreness and aches from being in bed when one is not used to it.

My complaints were taken seriously, and everything possible was done to ease the soreness. I had been in the hospital about a week when the doctor cleared out a small wing and put me in there by myself. He kept me there just as long as he possibly could without inconvenience to other patients. It was quieter. Noise did bother me a little bit.

Someway, I found that I was very fortunate when I got to talking to the nurses and the others that I came in contact with, for I found that many of them had greater problems than I to wrestle with. The tenth day the doctor began to get me out of the oxygen tent, and within a couple of days I could dispense with it completely. I was glad to get rid of it, though I realize it eased my breathing during the necessary period and I am grateful for it. It was then that I learned that I had been on the critical list all that time. I hadn't realized that I was in any danger, and I felt like someone had just given me some sort of a renewed lease.

About this time I received a bit of additional education and a couple of new words for my vocabulary. They told me I was now suffering from a 'myocardial infarction.' I couldn't even pronounce it. I was impressed. The doctor explained that once there was a clot blocking an artery in the heart, that particular branch of the artery was no longer usable and there was an area of damage around the clot that was the infarction. This was the thing that would take so long to heal and render me almost immobile for months to come.

And out of this has come the really great trials in the entire ordeal. There is the everlasting waiting and resting. There is the frustration of finding that you really can't endure any amount of activity. I suppose this is worse for a person in middle life than for a person in his sixties, seventies, or eighties. At any rate, I have suffered an irony of ambition versus performance, for I find my mind racing with new projects and my body unable to perform a tenth of the activity my mind impatiently calls for.

I have the most patient of doctors. He explains everything in detail and answers my questions very completely and honestly. I respect the disease, but I am not now particularly apprehensive about it any more than I am apprehensive about riding downtown in the car. I accept the fact that there are many automobile accidents, my driver may have one before we reach our destination, and I may be killed. I take every precaution against this, but I don't necessarily think that it will happen to me on this trip. I don't stop riding in automobiles. I find that I have about the same plans and ambitions for the future that I always had.

Came the day when the ward became so crowded it was necessary to move me back into a room where there were about 35 other patients. I noticed the little inconveniences and annoyances all right. But by this time I was a lot more concerned about going home. This became my all-consuming objective.

I was confined to the hospital and that one bed for a month. It has now been 3 months since I got home, and I have still not been able to return to work. But my activity is increasing, and I am feeling better daily.

As I think back about my hospital experience, it was a real adventure. I met a new kind of people to me. I live in a striving climate in my work, and in the hospital staff I found people who were not striving for anything beyond helping other people. I admire them tremendously. They were very kind and considerate not only of me but of all those around me.

I liked the hospital's liberal policy about having company. It might have bothered other patients, but speaking for myself, company had a cheering effect. Nurses showed concern far beyond actual duties, accepting me as a special project—traveling clear across town to get me literature about coronary diseases. So I had all the information I wanted about the disease.

I pace myself differently now and am determined to do nothing that will contribute to another attack. I have had one slight one since getting out of the hospital. I simply overestimated my strength and didn't realize it until too late. I am a great deal more careful now.

A coronary thrombosis is a maturing experience. You get to feeling quite mature in a matter of minutes—that 90-year-old feeling. But that passes. The maturity that does not pass, however, is a new realization of really important things. It's sobering but rewarding, if one can but forget his knocking knees and chattering teeth and look for the bright side."

One of the messages Mr. Rodgers conveys is his attempts to stay in control of the situation and remain independent. He communicates ways in which he tried to give himself support, both physically and emotionally, until other support systems were made available. He clearly portrays the double bind he experienced between his mental desires and his physical capabilities. Self-centeredness, generally associated with illness, was described and identified by Mr. Rodgers when he told his wife he might not make it home, even though he knew this might worry her. Denial of illness and rationalization are evident throughout his description of the experience. Long-range goals were forced to be stored in exchange for more realistic short-term goals. He gradually but reluctantly began to accept a change in his life-style. He clearly describes his reaction to the repetitive and exhaustive questioning by hospital personnel in the health care facility. These are but a few of the insights provided from the client serving as teacher. The reader is encouraged to further explore his messages and their meaning in light of nursing intervention.

SUGGESTED BIBLIOGRAPHY

Bruner, Jerome S.: *Toward a Theory of Instruction*, The Belknap Press of Harvard University Press, Cambridge, Mass., 1975.
Cooper, Signe Skott: *Contemporary Nursing Practice: A Guide for the Returning Nurse*, McGraw-Hill Book Co., New York, 1970.
———— and May Shiga Hornback: *Continuing Nursing Education*, McGraw-Hill Book Co., New York, 1973.
Mager, Robert F.: *Preparing Instructional Objectives*, 2d ed., Fearon Publishers, Belmont, Calif., 1975.
Pluckhan, Margaret L., Sister Regina Peltier, and Elizabeth Spicher: "Meeting the Challenge: Coordination and Facilitation of Statewide Continuing Education for Nurses through Interdisciplinary and Interagency Action," *Journal of Continuing Education in Nursing*, 4 (1):22–27, January–February 1973.
Pohl, Margaret L.: *The Teaching Function of the Nursing Practitioner*, 2d ed., Wm. C. Brown Co., Publishers, Dubuque, Iowa, 1973.

Chapter 11

Management

If you have developed the ability to handle people, you don't need anything else. If you have not developed that ability, it doesn't matter much what else you have.

Anonymous

One of man's most characteristic functions is that of building systems of communication. A prime objective of management must be to establish and maintain an effective communication system that can assure that accurate, comprehensive, current, and appropriate data will be available for making organizational decisions. A study of the internal communication patterns within an organization and the external patterns of communication with other agencies provides valuable clues as to the functioning of that organization.

    Management involves converting information into action. It requires the marshaling of resources, particularly human resources, to accomplish that purpose. The organization must be so designed that management can orchestrate the application of skills and energies of those diverse individuals and groups within it to function as an integrated whole. If the organization cannot do that, there is no need for it because its goals can then be attained by individuals functioning alone.

There are managers at all levels of any organization. All professional nurses function in some managerial capacity within some communication network in the organization in which they are employed. The team leader is a manager of the personnel assigned to the team. The communication skills needed by the team leader are essentially the same as those required by the director of nursing service or dean of a school of nursing. The team leader allocates resources based on the judgment he or she makes about client needs and then matches team members' capabilities with those client needs. By placing the right person on the right job, the team leader blends and optimizes the skills of all members toward meeting a mutual goal of care.

A discussion of the many ways in which communication and management are in juxtaposition with one another would require a book in itself. Only a few of these can be presented here, primarily as examples.

THE PHILOSOPHY OF MANAGMENT

The approaches the manager uses and the outcomes he expects as he manages human resources depend to a large degree upon his general philosophy about those resources. McGregor[1] developed his theory X and theory Y as reflections of opposing assumptions about human nature and behavior. *Theory X* proposes that the average human being has an inherent dislike for work and will avoid it whenever possible. He needs to be controlled and threatened with punishment in efforts to motivate him to perform. It is assumed that individuals have little ambition and prefer being directed rather than taking responsibility on their own. *Theory Y*, on the other hand, assumes that people do *not* inherently dislike work and in fact find work a source of satisfaction. Individuals are highly imaginative and creative and exercise self-direction and self-control. It is obvious that whichever philosophy is held by the manager will be reflected in the communication behavior he displays towards those individuals for whom he is responsible.

The managerial symbols of "the carrot and the stick" represent dichotomous approaches to motivating individuals to use their potential. The "carrot" is the enticing positive reward approach, while the "stick" is the punitive method used in motivating individuals to perform. The verbal message of the former would be "If you do . . .," while the latter's mes-

[1]Douglas McGregor, *The Human Side of Enterprise,* McGraw-Hill Book Co., New York, 1960.

sage would be "If you don't. . . ." Again the managerial climate and communication between manager and employee would depend upon some basic assumptions of the manager regarding the general nature of employees.

Many people believe strongly in the Peter principle, which states that in a hierarchy every employee tends to rise to his level of incompetence.[2] There is a less well-known principle that managers must also consider as they strive to utilize human resources within organizations. It may be called the "Paul principle." It states that for every employee who rises *above* his level of competence, there are several whose full talents are never fully utilized. The waste in manpower and ability is deplorable. Again, that 85 percent of every person's unused potential that lies dormant in each of us must be tapped and put to use. Many employees have never even been allowed to fail because they have never been allowed to take on added responsibility. It was only by a stroke of fate that a haberdasher from Missouri, Harry S. Truman, became not only our 32nd President but also possibly one of the greatest of all times.

The communication breakdown experienced in many organizations is due to the fact that healthy dialogue, the open and effective form of interpersonal communication, is not congruent with the concept of so many social organizations in which hierarchical structures operate. The communication patterns of stable individuals and stable organizations have much in common. Dialogical relationships require the mutual giving and receiving of information freely and openly. Individuals at various levels in any organization cannot function when others seek to control and/or distort the information needed to carry out their responsibility.

COMMUNICATION NETWORKS

The effective and efficient flow of information throughout an organization, whether focusing on the nursing team, the nursing service, or the entire health team, depends upon the communication networks that have been established. *Formal communication networks* generally are expected to follow organizational lines, be fluid, and flow in all directions. The *organizational chart*, which displays the placement of departments, positions, and/or individuals to one another, should indicate the actual flow of communication within the agency. However, in studying many organizations in which communication problems exist, it is not uncommon to find little similarity between the actual flow of information and the organizational structure, or between what is verbalized as networks used and what exists

[2]Lawrence J. Peter and Raymond Hull, *The Peter Principle,* William Morrow, New York, 1969.

in reality. The speed as well as the accuracy with which information flows through the system for decision making are critical factors. Having too many supervisors along the pathways may impede the flow of data.

Many formal communication networks become sluggish, clogged, and dysfunctional to some individuals along the pathways. When this happens, collateral support systems, much like the collateral blood supplies that develop to assist dysfunctional circulatory networks, develop to supply the information needed. These *informal communication networks* are commonly called *grapevines*, and they carry the messages labeled *rumors*. Some people believe that grapevines are a normal part of all communication systems. However, it is generally found that the degree to which they are present bears a direct relationship to the ineffectiveness of formal channels in handling the information flow. Grapevines and rumors are often viewed as symptomatic of communication breakdown within an organization. They may be indicative of ineffective and/or excessive number of circuits through which information must flow. They may reflect the unconscious or intentional withholding of information from individuals who believe they need that information. The informal networks may be a blessing in disguise, for they may be responsible for keeping an organization's communication lifeline open and viable.

There is a tendency for the information that flows through informal channels to be distorted because the voids have often been filled with inferences rather than facts, assumptions instead of realities, and expectations instead of truths. For example, as one individual at one end of the grapevine said to another, "I won't go into all the details; in fact, I've already told you more about it than I heard myself."

Distrust often breeds and nourishes rumors. If individuals in the organization are suspicious of the data being sent and feel that there may be hidden agendas, information will be distorted. Rumors, like the graffiti on restroom walls, serve as a sort of catharsis. Too often, the administration's concern centers on identifying *where* the rumor or misinformation started rather than studying the reasons *why* it began. The latter approach would generally uncover some inadequacies within the formal communication system of the organization.

SOME MANAGEMENT PRINCIPLES

The following four general management principles are presented as a means of showing various ways in which human communication is involved in management.

Span of control relates to the size of the group or number of individuals a manager has in his area of control and responsibility. There is an obvious limit to the size of the human resources—the number of employees—a person can effectively manage. As each member is added to a group, the number of potential interpersonal communication exchanges increases geometrically, not arithmetically. The potential for interpersonal relationship problems would increase for the manager in the same way. Therefore the manager's span of control, or number of individuals under his control, must be a prime consideration in planning the organizational structure if effective management is desired.

Consultive management is the democratic approach of involving group members in the decision-making process. It helps foster feelings of belongingness, identity, and ownership, which relate to personal needs and often serve as motivations to increase productivity. When managers solicit ideas and suggestions from the employees within the organization, not only are valuable inputs for problem solving provided but also a sense of worth, trust, confidence, and respect is communicated to the members. However, this healthy psychological climate will be destroyed if the employees do not receive *feedback* regarding the use of their ideas. More damage can be done to the esprit de corps within an organization if ideas are solicited but never really considered in the decision-making process than if they had never been requested.

Unity of command relates to the fact that an individual cannot be answerable to more than one manager at a time. Some organizational structures are so ill-conceived as to place employees in double bind positions in which they receive incongruent messages and commands. It is analogous to the situation of a child who receives one message of how to behave from the mother and a totally different and often opposite message from the father. Confusion, frustration, and hostility often result.

Authority must be commensurate with responsibility. All too frequently, individuals have been assigned the responsibility to accomplish a designated task but have not been given the needed authority with which to fulfill that commitment. Their situation is analogous to the untenable position of a police officer who is responsible for catching criminals, yet has no authority or laws to support him. Verbal directives take on meaning in relation to how much authority the sender is perceived to have to enforce them. The individual who has responsibility but lacks the accompanying authority is frustrated and often demoralized when placed in that position.

The subject of evaluation, whether performance evaluation or assessment of quality of care, is an important concern of management in health care delivery systems. Evaluation is basically a communication *feedback* process that must be continuous.

The term *performance* evaluation is preferable to *personnel* evaluation because it should help to place the emphasis where it belongs: on the *behavior*, not the *person*. Antecedent to performance evaluation, the philosophy, goals, and expectations of management must be clearly developed and communicated to those working in the organization. All too often, individuals accept employment in agencies in which their personal and/or professional goals are at odds with the organizational goals; rewards are not given for behavior they expected to be rewarded. It is not until months later, when problems develop and/or their performance is evaluated formally, that the disparity in goals and expectations is realized. Kramer[3] discussed the *reality shock* experienced by the neophyte nurses employed in hospital settings, who have programmed professional values that are not in concert with the experienced reality of the work setting.

Communication skills in the hands of directors of nursing, supervisors, head nurses, team leaders, faculty, and all others involved are essential if performance evaluation is to have a positive effect on motivation, growth, and learning. Too often it is perceived and communicated as a punitive process rather than a helping one.

In our "era of accountability" in health care delivery, when supporting data are required to justify our existence, means of assessment must continuously be addressed. Individuals in the field must be skilled in communicating the need for health care programs to the public—the consumers of those services. The philosophy behind zero-base budgeting, adopted by the Carter administration, requires that priorities of programming be established with the accompanying budgetary requests. The intrapersonal thought processing used in making choices and the interpersonal relationships established to gain group consensus will require communication skill.

The medical profession is involved in assessing the quality of care. The Professional Standards Review Organizations (PSROs) were established by law as the medical profession's evaluating mechanism. All health care providers are becoming increasingly involved in making evaluations to provide data to consumers regarding the quality of care given.

LEADERSHIP OR SUPERVISION

Leadership *and* supervision are terms generally associated with the topic of management. Both involve interpersonal communication and relate to ways of influencing people. Endless numbers of studies have been and are being conducted to identify the styles, traits, behavior, and functions of leadership and the characteristics of supervision.

Dansereau et al.[4] used a less traditional approach in their study, which

[3]Marlene Kramer, *Reality Shock: Why Nurses Leave Nursing,* C. V. Mosby Co., St. Louis, 1974.

[4]Fred Dansereau Jr., George Graen, and William J. Haga, "A Vertical Dyad Linkage Approach to Leadership within Formal Organizations: A Longitudinal Investigation of the Role Making Process," *Organizational Behavior and Human Performance,* **13**: 46–78, 1975.

was based on earlier works of Jacobs,[5] to uncover some of the "mysteries" of the leadership phenomenon. They considered leadership and supervision as parallel phenomenons that differed in the use of authority by the superior. The superior always has the authority but *leadership* exchanges involve influence *without* the use of authority while *supervision* involves influence based primarily upon the use of authority.[6]

   This theory is worthy of investigation because the communication exchange lies at the core of the difference between leadership and supervision, which are viewed as techniques used to influence. Concern is for each individual dyadic relationship, that of the superior and each linking member, in the group. This theory does not consider the relationship between the superior and the group as a whole. Superiors typically employ *both* leadership and supervision techniques. Members of each dyad are interdependent, and the communication pattern depends upon both members of each dyad. When using the *supervision technique*, the superior relies almost exclusively on the formal employment contract, rules, and regulations in dealing with the member, who has subscribed to those rules as a condition of employment and is compensated for submitting to that authority. The superior using *leadership techniques* does not rely exclusively on the contract even though he has the authority to do so. He exerts influence through an interpersonal-exchange relationship. Each linking member is involved actively in decision making and has ready access to information. Confidence and consideration are shown to the member who reciprocates with more highly valued output. Both members of the dyad make a commitment and assume responsibility. The superior is highly dependent upon the other member of the dyad. If at any time of interaction with the member, supervision is used to solve problems, it would damage the leadership relationship. The superior allows more freedom for the member in negotiating job-related matters than would the superior using supervision techniques. While supervision relies on rules and compliance, leadership influences through interpersonal commitment. From the Dansereau et al. study,[7] it was concluded that an organization, department, or unit needs an appropriate mix of dyads in which some members need and receive leadership and others receive supervision. They stated that "Although the management of an organizational unit clearly involves dealing with the entire set of members, leadership can only occur in the vertical dyad."[8] Each member of the dyad must be considered individually. Some

---

[5]T. Jacobs, *Leadership and Exchange in Formal Research Organizations*, Human Resources Organization, Alexandria, Va., 1971.

[6]Dansereau, Jr., et al., "A Vertical Dyad Linkage Approach to Leadership within Formal Organizations," p. 48.

[7]Dansereau, Jr., et al., "A Vertical Dyad Linkage Approach to Leadership within Formal Organizations."

[8]Dansereau, Jr., et al. "A Vertical Dyad Linkage Approach to Leadership within Formal Organizations," p. 76.

members are obviously not ready and/or willing to take responsibility, to make a commitment to the organization, or to develop ownership feelings created by leadership techniques of the superior.

There are numerous ways to view the philosophy and principles of management as well as to study leadership and supervision. However, irrespective of the approach used, the communication behavior of the manager at all levels of the organization must be considered. We can take little consolation in knowing that health care organizations are not unique in their bureacratic red tape and ineptness. It would seem that as members of a human service organization, we should be the first to exemplify a truly humanistic approach to management.

SUGGESTED BIBLIOGRAPHY

Baker, Frank, Peter J. M. McEwan, and Alan Sheldon (eds.): *Industrial Organizations and Health Vol. 1: Selected Readings*, Tavistock Publications, New York, 1969.

Blau, Peter M.: *On the Nature of Organizations*, John Wiley & Sons, New York, 1974.

Bormann, Ernest G., William S. Howell, Ralph G. Nichols, and George L. Shapiro: *Interpersonal Communication in the Modern Organization*, Prentice-Hall, Englewood Cliffs, N.J., 1969.

Brown, Barbara J.: "The Role of Nursing Administrator in Patient Care Delivery Systems," *Nursing Administration Quarterly*, 1(1):1–6, Fall 1976.

Donovan, Helen, M.: *Nursing Service Administration: Managing the Enterprise*, C. V. Mosby Co., St. Louis, 1975.

Douglass, Laura Mae and EM Olivia Bevis: *Nursing Leadership in Action: Principles and Application to Staff Situations*, 2d ed., C. V. Mosby Co., St. Louis, 1974.

Etzioni, Amitai: *Modern Organizations*, Prentice-Hall, Englewood Cliffs, N.J., 1964.

Leininger, Madeline: "The Leadership Crisis in Nursing: A Critical Problem and Challenge," *Journal of Nursing Administration,* 4(2):28–34, March–April 1974.

McGregor, Douglas: *The Human Side of Enterprise*, McGraw-Hill Book Co., New York, 1960.

Pyhrr, Peter A.: "Zero-Base Budgeting," *Harvard Business Review,* 48:111–121, November–December 1970.

Schein, Edgar H.: *Organizational Psychology*, Prentice-Hall, Englewood Cliffs, N.J., 1965.

Stewart, Charles J. and William B. Cash: *Interviewing: Principles and Practices*, Wm. C. Brown Co., Publishers, Dubuque, Iowa, 1974.

Vardaman, George T. and Carroll C. Halterman: *Managerial Control through Communication: Systems for Organizational Diagnosis and Design*, John Wiley & Sons, New York, 1968.

Chapter 12

The Process of Change

Not everything that is faced can be changed, but nothing can be changed until it is faced.

James Baldwin

Change is an essential part of both our personal and our professional lives. We live in a fluid, not static, world where change is inevitable. One need only to scan any daily newspaper to find numerous articles that report changes that will affect health care either directly or indirectly. For organizations to remain viable, they must have not only a *maintenance function* but also an *innovative function* to adapt to a continuously changing world. Today's facts become tomorrow's misinformation. As Will Rogers once said, "It's not what I don't know that gets me in trouble, it's the things I know that aren't so." The play entitled *Stop the World I Want to Get Off* reflects the desire of many individuals who are frustrated with the speed of change. *Future shock* was the label Toffler[1] assigned to the

[1]Toffler, *Future Shock*.

increasing lag between the pace of environmental change and the limited pace of human response to it.

COMMUNICATION AND CHANGE

There would be no change, no progress, in fact, no civilized life as we know it today without human communication. The process of change is embedded in our intrapersonal and interpersonal communication behavior.

Change begins with our intrapersonal *thought process*. It is here where new ways of ordering and structuring our world are developed and new ideas and approaches formulated. Change is also intimately related to the intrapersonal communication process when *external inputs interface with one's internally stored program*. The brain has its own laws that dictate if and how new symbolic inputs will be processed. The process is displayed in the intrapersonal communication model (Figure 2-2) presented in Chapter 2. We structure incoming messages around the unique internal program we have spent a lifetime creating out of our unique experiences. In varying degree we spend the rest of our lives defending it from discrepant inputs.

Through interpersonal communication we are apprised of the fact that the world *we* have created is not the *only* world. As we communicate with others and are *influenced by them*, we are made aware of differences in perception and are forced to question our programmed system of values and beliefs. As Barnlund said, "No one can leave the safety and comfort of his own assumptive world and enter that of another without running the risk of having his own commitments questioned."[2] The interpersonal exchange forces us to resolve the conflict, or dissonance, and to free ourselves from the tension and discomfort it has caused. When we communicate with others, we are always vulnerable to being influenced to accept a new way of viewing the world and adapt to change. We may, however, communicate with others to get the support we need to discard or distort external inputs that are not in accord with the data in our internal storage.

Most of our interpersonal communication is centered around change—around trying to influence others to accept our ideas and our products or services; to share our feelings, values, and view of the world. As nurses, we help clients cope by changing their perception of their illness and its treatment. We help them learn and accept a new life-style that is more in concert with their abilities. Through interpersonal communication, we serve as *change agents* and *catalysts of change* to maintain a viable health care delivery system.

[2]Barnlund, "Communication: The Context of Change," p. 37.

THE CHANGE PROCESS

It is human nature to get into ruts and routine ways of behaving, into patterned and habitual responses. But the status quo, while safe and comfortable, has no place in a dynamic world. The explanation for our resistance to change can be found in the intrapersonal communication process, in which we have the need to maintain internal consistency and resist inputs that we cannot make conform to the data already stored.

Individuals vary in their ability to accommodate dissonant data and change their internal belief system. Harvey[3] described the System IV abstract individuals as flexible, adaptable, creative, and open to change. Unfortunately, our world consists of predominantly System I individuals, who are concrete and rigid. These are the individuals whose minds are like cement—all mixed up and permanently set! Dogmatism, or closed-mindedness, is one of the greatest deterrents to change. Those who resist change frequently defend their actions with such statements as "It's a foolish idea and won't work," "It's not a bad idea, but this isn't the right time," "The time is ripe, but we couldn't work out that idea here," and finally, "I really favored the idea from the beginning." These are attempts to save face.

Experiencing incongruent messages can be a painful yet necessary ingredient for initiating change. Tension, anxiety, and discomfort provide the motivating force that results in individuals' willingness to give up even their most highly prized values. Sometimes individuals are not ready for change because they do not feel they have the capacity for other ways of behaving. Others can help motivate individuals to change, but the change must be made by each individual himself.

Without some pain, there may be no gains, no chance to grow. Having lived as a vegetarian and a teetotaler for 60 years, a Swiss "Peace Apostle," Max Daetwyler, was asked why he had started eating meat and drinking wine at age 80. He defended his change of mind by saying, "Only fools insist on errors." So it is with individuals who have their foot on the brake to stop changes in their lives and try to keep the status quo. The mind is like an umbrella: it doesn't work unless it is open!

Change involves *taking risks* whether in oneself adapting to change, influencing others to change, or initiating change in a health care system. Change requires being deviant and innovative. In trying out new ideas there are bound to be failures. Yet society does not look well on failures. Nurses as a group have not been oriented and acculturated to be good risk takers. Assertiveness training and other means have been used to help

[3]O. J. Harvey, "System Structure, Flexibility, and Creativity," in O. J. Harvey (ed)., *Experience, Structure and Adaptability,* Springer, New York, 1966, 39–65.

improve one's self-concept and security in an effort to increase one's willingness to take risks.

We can never learn unless we try. Unless we are willing to take risks, make changes, and have support in doing it, we stay where we are. Referring to the study by Dansereau et al., they found that "Without a good deal of confidence that one's superior will support innovative approaches to problems and tasks on the job, the assumption of such risk as an exercise of latitude is not likely to occur."[4] They concluded that the leadership technique would be amenable to fostering change.

Students and faculty in nursing programs often serve as successful change agents as they influence the direction of health care. Support, sanction, and rewards must be given for innovation and initiating change. The federal dollar is one of our most effective change agents, probably because the reward is worth the risk of change.

In many ways the turtle might be considered symbolic of change. Like the turtle, one does not get anywhere unless he takes risks and sticks his neck out. The hard shell of the turtle is needed to withstand the knocks and discomfort associated with change. We need a good many more turtles in the nursing profession to keep pace with the rapid changes we are experiencing in health care today. Each individual is his own reservoir of motivation and change. Change and new ideas will be accompanied by failures as well as successes. It might be well to recall the successes and positive approach of the great inventor Thomas A. Edison. He is said to have tried 50,000 different combinations before coming up with a successful new storage battery. Asked if that wasn't a big waste of time, he replied, "Nonsense. I now know 50,000 things that won't work."

SUGGESTED BIBLIOGRAPHY

Bennis, Warren G., Kenneth D. Benne, Robert Chin, and Kenneth E. Corey: *The Planning of Change*, 3d ed., Holt Rinehart & Winston, New York, 1976.

Harvey, O. J.: "Conceptual Systems and Attitude Change," in Carolyn W. Sherif and Muzafer Sherif (eds.), *Attitude, Ego-Involvement and Change*, John Wiley & Sons, New York, 1967, pp. 201–226.

Munn, Yvonne L.: "Power: How to Get it and Use it in Nursing Today," *Nursing Administration Quarterly*, 1(1):95–103, Fall 1976.

Patton, Bobby R. and Kim Giffin: *Problem-Solving Group Interaction*, Harper & Row, Publishers, New York, 1973.

[4]Dansereau, Jr., et al., "A Vertical Dyad Linkage Approach to Leadership within Formal Organization," p. 71.

Tobin, Helen M., Pat S. Yoder, Peggy K. Hull, and Barbara Clark Scott: *The Process of Staff Development: Components for Change*, C. V. Mosby Co., St. Louis, 1974.

White, B. J. and O. J. Harvey: "Effects of Personality and Own Stand on Judgment and Production of Statements about a Central Issue," *Journal of Experimental Social Psychology*, I:334–347, 1965.

Chapter 13

Et Cetera

Books are but waste paper unless we spend in action the wisdom we get from thought.

Bulwer

It seems appropriate to conclude this manuscript with a basic principle from the field of general semantics—*etc.*—the symbol that admits the fact that, try as we might, we could never say all about anything! There is always more that could have been written—about other theories, principles, and methodologies. An infinite number of areas of nursing practice in which communication skills are needed could have been presented. Even though the functional areas that were selected were presented by way of example, injustice has been done, for example, to the all-important area of scientific study. Human communication enters into all phases of *research*, from ideation and design of the study to gathering and processing of the data and eventual dissemination and diffusion of the findings in the field of practice. *Continuing education*, which reflects our concern for keeping a current and comprehensive information storage bank, was slighted, especially in view of its importance in nursing today. Only brief reference was made to *performance evaluation* and areas of *quality assessment*, which again require communication skill in the selection and processing of data. Presentation of some of the creative and exciting new approaches to *problem solving* must be shelved until some other time. One is reminded of a similar frustration voiced by Robert Frost in his poem "Mending Wall." He said, "Something there is that doesn't love a wall, . . . Before I built a wall I'd ask to know/what I was walling in or walling out." So it is with this manuscript, where the process of selecting what was to be "walled in" resulted in an automatic decision of what had to be "walled out."

As with our mind-body processes, the human communication process is but one more marvel, and to some extent a mystery, of mankind. It seems such a simple request to ask that the sender's messages and their intended meaning be at least to a degree congruent with the message meaning received. Yet the inherent mysteries associated with the communication process leave the answer to that request one of probabilities rather than certainties. As Pierce expressed the dilemma, "We have learned some remarkable things, but chiefly we live and communicate not through our understanding of these processes but in spite of our ignorances concerning them."[1]

Communication touches our personal and professional lives in a variety of interesting ways. Some of the ways we do not yet understand, some ways we fail to accept, and some remain out of our conscious awareness. Communication permeates every moment of our lives. There is no greater human malady than the loss of the ability to communication with ourselves, through mental illness, or of the opportunity to communicate with others, through isolation or confinement.

We create our own reality, and it is a galaxy of symbols. We continuously strive to make sense of that world, to communicate with the world, and to influence others. Each of us is a novel and interesting being, with a unique frame of reference that serves as the base from which we communicate. As Jean-Jacques Rousseau said: "I am not made like anyone I have ever seen. I dare believe that I am not made like anyone in existence. If I am not better, at least I am different."

Knowledge and understanding of the parameters of the process of human communication, as presented in Part I, are not enough, but admittedly are a good beginning to improving our communication behavior. It would be as foolhardy to expect one to become skilled as a communicator merely by knowing the concepts as it would be to expect an army private to be an expert marksman by knowing the parts of the M-16 rifle. The prime responsibility resides in the hands of the individual, who must apply the

[1]John R. Pierce, "Communications," *Scientific American,* **227**(3):31, September 1972.

knowledge through practice and experiences in the daily management of his personal and professional lives.

While the human communication game is a gamble, a game of chance, it is a game of life that must be played. Efforts must be continuously directed toward improving our odds as we seek to match the meaning of messages. There is no more worthy challenge or greater reward for those who are willing to spend the time and effort to improve their communication behavior. The comprehensive study of human communication is a Herculean task, for it involves an infinite number of areas of concern: verbal and nonverbal language, theories of personality, group dynamics, etc.,

etc.,

etc.

SUGGESTED BIBLIOGRAPHY

Pierce, John R.: "Communication," *Scientific American*, **227**(3):31–41, September 1972.

Index